75

TREATMENT OF
MULTIPLE PERSONALITY DISORDER

TREATMENT OF
MULTIPLE PERSONALITY DISORDER

Edited by

Bennett G. Braun, M.D.
Director, Dissociative Disorders Program,
Rush-Presbyterian-St. Luke's Medical Center,
Rush University, Chicago;
Director, Associated Mental Health Services, Chicago

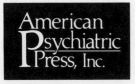

American Psychiatric Press, Inc.
Washington, D.C.

Library of Congress Cataloging in Publication Data

Main entry under title:

Treatment of multiple personality disorder.

 Includes bibliographies.
 1. Multiple personality in children—Treatment.
2. Psychotherapy. 3. Multiple personality in children—Chemotherapy.
I. Braun, Bennett G. II. Title: Childhood antecedents of multiple
personality. [DNLM: 1. Multiple-Personality Disorder—therapy. WM
173.6 T784]
RJ506.M84C48   1985   Suppl   616.92′85236   86-10903
ISBN 0-88048-096-3 (soft : alk. paper)

DEDICATION

This work is dedicated to the people who have had a major
positive impact on my professional development
(in chronological order):

Thelma H. Braun and Milton L. Braun, D.D.S.
Arthur L. Irion, Ph.D.
My patients
Jan Fawcett, M.D.
Robert J. Kearney, Ph.D.
Jane E. Braun, M.Ed.

Contents

Contributors

ROBERT BARKIN, M.B.A., PHARM.D.
Assistant Director, Pharmacy, Rush-Presbyterian-St. Luke's Medical Center, Chicago; Faculty, Department of Pharmacology, Rush Medical College; Faculty, Department of Pharmaceuticals, College of Pharmacy, University of Illinois at Chicago

BENNETT G. BRAUN, M.D.
Instructor, Department of Psychiatry, Rush Medical College; Director, Dissociative Disorders Program, Rush-Presbyterian-St. Luke's Medical Center, Rush University; Adjunct Associate Professor, Department of Psychology, University of Illinois at Chicago; Director, Associated Mental Health Services

DAVID CAUL, M.D.
Director, Southeastern Ohio Institute for the Diagnosis and Treatment of Multiple Personality

RICHARD P. KLUFT, M.D.
Assistant Clinical Professor of Psychiatry, Temple University School of Medicine; Attending Psychiatrist, The Institute of the Pennsylvania Hospital, Philadelphia; Visiting Associate Professor, Department of Psychiatry, Rush Medical College, Chicago

FRANK W. PUTNAM, M.D.
Neuropsychiatry Branch, National Institute of Mental Health, St. Elizabeths Hospital, Washington, D.C.

ROBERTA G. SACHS, PH.D.
Research Consultant, Dissociative Disorders Program, Rush-Presbyterian-St. Luke's Medical Center, Rush University, Chicago

DAVID SPIEGEL, M.D.
*Associate Professor of Psychiatry and Behavioral Sciences
(Clinical) and Director of the Adult Psychiatric Outpatient Clinic,
Stanford University School of Medicine, Stanford, California*

CORNELIA B. WILBUR, M.D.
*Professor Emeritus, University of Kentucky College of Medicine;
Attending Psychiatrist, Good Samaritan Hospital, Lexington,
Kentucky*

Introduction

Throughout most of the 20th century, until about a decade ago, only an occasional single paper appeared on multiple personality disorder (MPD) in scientific literature. Discussions were so rare that little or no continuity was established to lay a basis for conceptualization of MPD as anything other than what it was generally thought to be: clinical oddity, historical curiosity, or hoax.

Unless the reader is thoroughly familiar with recent scientific literature on MPD, his or her approach to this book may be colored to some extent by the ubiquitous popular literature on the subject. Multiple personality also is a much-used—often misused—device in fiction, theater, and television. The phenomenology of MPD that emerges from scientific and clinical observation is not necessarily reflected accurately by the craft of the journalist or the art of the playwright.

A brief overview of current concepts of multiplicity may be helpful to the reader who is approaching the subject in scientific light for the first time.

Braun (1980, 1984b) described MPD as the demonstration in one person of two or more personalities, each of whom possesses identifiably distinctive, consistently ongoing characteristics and a relatively separate memory of individual life history. Executive control of the body is transferred from one personality to another, but the total individual is never out of touch with reality. Some or all of the personalities frequently experience periods of amnesia, time loss, or blackouts. Amnesia for thoughts and actions of other personalities often occurs in the host personality, which is the one who has executive control of the body the greatest percentage of the time during a given time period. What appear to be auditory hallucinations consisting of comments on activities or thoughts and feelings of being influenced are common. These are manifestations of personalities' being aware of thoughts and actions of other personalities who are not in control or who are not co-conscious.

The word *personality* is used often in this book, so the basic definition of this and other terms used in the MPD literature should be established:

Personality—an entity that has the following: a) a consistent and ongoing set of response patterns to given stimuli; b) a significant confluent history; c) a range of emotions available (anger, sadness, joy, and so on); and d) a range of intensity of affect for each emotion (for example, anger ranging from neutrality to frustration and irritation to anger and rage).

The concept of MPD is easier to comprehend when the personalities are perceived as thought processes with their concomitant physiological processes separated by repression barriers of sorts. It also might become a more understandable illness, and therefore more accepted, if the numbers of personalities were not alleged to be so great. It is difficult to conceive of a patient's having 40 or more full personalities; a patient's having several personalities and many fragments makes more sense. Fragments require less interaction and intensity of therapy prior to integration.

Fragment—an entity that is less than a personality. Fragments have a consistent and ongoing set of response patterns to given stimuli and either a significant history or a range of emotions/affect, but usually not both to the same degree. For example, in one patient a fragment was created to express frustration and anger for the system; it had a long life history and a full range of anger, but could express or experience little sadness or joy. Another patient had a fragment with a minimal life history but a full range of emotions: This fragment was created to deal with in-laws who were intensely disliked by the host personality. Though most all emotions were present and could vary in intensity, this fragment's life history consisted only of experiences when the family got together on holidays and for occasional weddings and funerals.

Special-purpose fragment—an entity that is less than a fragment. It has a limited set of response patterns to stimuli and minimal life history and range of emotion/affect. For example, the function of one fragment in a patient was to perform fellatio; this was in response to the patient's being whipped and forced to perform fellatio on her brother for child pornography. Another named Melody expressed the thoughts of others through music. (Names often have special significance and these patients often "talk" in coded language.)

Memory trace fragment—a fragment that has only a minimal set of response patterns to stimuli, life history, and range of emotion/affect but has knowledge for a short period of time. This is to be differentiated from a *memory trace personality* (Dr. Cornelia Wilbur, personal communication, May 1979), which has knowledge of the entire life experience of the multiple.

Alter (also called *alternate personality*)—any personality or fragment other than the host personality.

Host personality—the personality that has executive control of the body for the greatest percentage of time during a given time period. For example, in one patient, Sally had control from birth until age 3, when Sarah took over and was out 60 percent of the time. At age 7, a specific trauma occurred, and Hanna took over until puberty at age 12, when Roz became the host by being out 45 percent of the time, the rest of the time being shared among the others. From age 17 to the present, Joan has been the host personality.

Presenting personality—the entity that first comes in for therapy; it may be the original personality, the host personality, or a fragment.

Original personality—the entity that developed first after birth and split off or remained separate from the flow of the rest of the thought processes. The original personality is often difficult to locate and work with, but this needs to be done to achieve a stable and lasting integration.

Splitting—the creation of a new entity by the splitting off or coalescing of energy which forms the nucleus of a separate personality or fragment.

Switching—going back and forth between already existing personalities or fragments. This may be precipitated by external or internal stimuli.

Two-way amnesia—the state in which one personality or fragment does not know of the existence of another personality or fragment and vice versa.

One-way amnesia—the state in which personality/fragment A does not know anything about personality/fragment B, but B knows everything about A. Personality/fragment B is, so to speak, like a good "tail" who follows someone without being observed.

Co-presence—the simultaneous presence of two or more personalities/fragments with or without their knowing of one another's existence or current presence. Co-presence can occur with or without an influence of one upon another.

Co-consciousness—the state of being aware of the thoughts or consciousness of another personality. It can be unidirectional or bidirectional, with or without co-presence, and/or with or without an influence of one upon another.

Fusion—the act or instance of bringing together two or more personalities or fragments in order to blend their essence into a single entity. This is usually accompanied by some neuro-psychophysiologic signs.

Integration—the process of bringing together the separate thought processes (personalities or fragments) and maintaining them as

one. It is a process that starts before fusion and continues after
it.

Clinical manifestations of MPD can be perplexing and har-
rowing for the therapist. Switching of personalities may produce diverse physical appearances such as strikingly different
facial expressions, permutations in posture and body language,
change in handedness, different hair styles, reversals in out-
ward gender presentation, significant weight gain or loss over
short periods of time, and voice changes.

Alternate personalities may demonstrate the behaviors that
manifest their perceptions of themselves. They may speak in
different accents and even different languages; their hand-
writing may be different; some may be creative in different
arts, others not at all; and some may be male, others female in
their self-perceptions, life histories, and dress.

Some of the personalities may have psychophysiological
symptoms that are not experienced by others. The most frequently seen are headaches, anxiety manifestations, unpredictable responses to medication, chest pain, extreme sensitivity/
tolerance to pain, conversionlike symptoms, gastrointestinal
problems, seizure disorders, and allergies. The range and apparent severity of such symptoms may mislead diagnosticians
for years (Braun 1983, Putnam 1983). Putnam (1983, 1986)
reported an average time in the mental health system of 6.8
years from entry to proper diagnosis for MPD patients. I have
confirmed this in a study of 126 cases, finding 6.88 years (unpublished manuscript).

The differential diagnosis of MPD (Coons 1984) is also a list
of the various misdiagnoses. The disorders that a therapist may
consider include the organic, dissociative, substance abuse,
schizophrenic, paranoid, affective, anxiety, somatoform and
borderline personality disorders. Every diagnosis in the *Diagnostic and Statistical Manual of Mental Disorders* (*Third Edition*)
(*DSM–III;* American Psychiatric Association 1980) has at one
time or another been applied to MPD (Braun 1984b). The patient may actively resist diagnosis by withholding information
or lying or may guide the therapist in misdirections with con-
fabulation or by presenting knowledge (factual information
without affective component) as if it were full memory. It is not
unusual for the multiple personality patient to use knowledge/

memory confusions to camouflage amnesiac "missing time" (Braun 1985).

Multiple personality is a dissociative disorder and as such is characterized by a disruption of memory and identity. Funk and Wagnalls's *Standard College Dictionary* defines *dissociation* as "the process whereby a set of ideas, feelings, etc., loses most of its relationships with the rest of the personality, functioning somewhat independently." Braun (1985) proposed that the complex phenomena of dissociation can be conceptualized by the BASK model, which represents behavior, affect, sensation and knowledge functioning in parallel on a time continuum. The model permits graphic illustration of dissociative disorders, such as automatism (dissociation in behavior), hypnosis induced to create an anesthesia (dissociation in affect and sensation), and typical MPD (dissociation in all BASK elements). Consonant with the classic description of multiple personality, the MPD patient is never out of touch with reality because one or another of the personalities is always present with a more or less full range of BASK-encoded memory.

This book represents an initial advance toward the eventual preparation of a definitive work on the treatment of MPD. It lays the groundwork by presenting in print for the first time both the therapeutic work and the insights of clinicians and investigators, which heretofore were presented mainly in oral exchanges of information.

Publication of this book on treatment of MPD and a complementary work by Richard Kluft, *Childhood Antecedents to Multiple Personality* (1985) indicates the increase in clinical and research activity that has occurred since 1980, when MPD gained recognition in *DSM-III* as a dissociative disorder. The rediscovery of MPD as a mental disorder after decades of nonexistence in scientific and clinical thought has been chronicled in many publications and is referred to in several chapters in this monograph. Diagnosis of MPD by increasing numbers of clinicians has brought the total number of MPD patients from approximately 500 in 1979 (Braun 1980) to 1,000 in 1983 (Braun 1984a) to approximately 5,000 cases that I know of at the present time. This geometric increase has largely come about through the International Conference on Multiple Personality/Dissociative States sponsored annually by Rush–Presbyterian–St. Luke's Medical Center in Chicago. Empirical knowledge gained from diagnosing and treating increased numbers of MPD patients has contributed to formulation of theory regarding the etiology of MPD (Braun 1984b, Braun and Sachs 1985, Kluft 1984). And theory has helped to develop a better understanding of the disorder and dissociation in general.

In Chapter 1 of this book, I discuss two theoretical constructions of MPD and show how identification of the MPD patient's unique psychotherapeutic needs results from them. Both the 3-P (predisposing, precipitating, perpetuating factors) model of Braun and Sachs (1985) and the four-factor theory of Kluft (1984) place the following conditions at the center of the etiology of MPD: 1) high dissociative potential and ability to use dissociation as an ego defense and 2) childhood exposure to severe, repeated, and often bizarre physical, sexual, or emotional abuse that overwhelms the individual's defenses and is most often administered by parents or other family members who may irrationally intersperse abuse with expressions of love. In this chapter, 13 issues are discussed that the psychotherapist must address in undertaking treatment with the goal of integrating the patient's fragmented thought process.

In Chapter 2, Dr. Richard Kluft reviews his experience with 52 MPD patients and demonstrates that stable integration of personalities is possible, despite many difficulties that tend to promote relapse or incomplete integration. He shows that different factors promote relapse at different stages of the patient's path toward integration, from one week to 27 months. Nevertheless, MPD has an excellent prognosis if intense psychotherapy is available and the patient is willing to participate in the treatment.

Dr. David Spiegel, in Chapter 3, also emphasizes the etiological importance of dissociative potential and childhood history of severe repeated abuse by parents or family members who intersperse abuse with expressions of love. He sees this as a double bind of confusing messages inflicted on the patient: a primary injunction, a secondary injunction that contradicts the first, and an unspoken but powerfully enforced rule that the paradox cannot be openly addressed. The paradoxical communication demands that the patient act in two different ways at the same time. Dr. Spiegel proposes that MPD can be conceptualized as a posttraumatic stress disorder that arises in response to repeated double binding.

A 13-step plan for treatment of children with MPD is outlined
by Dr. Kluft in Chapter 4. Although most MPD patients are
adults, Dr. Kluft has knowledge of 50 child patients who are
under treatment by 20 different clinicians or investigators. He
demonstrates findings in MPD children that are largely consistent with the retrospective accounts of the genesis of MPD in
adult patients. In every instance in which treatment of a child
patient has been successful, the therapist has been able to effectively intervene to protect the child from further abuse. This
requires being able to relate to the various support systems in
the child's environment (e.g., parents; school administrators,
counselors, and teachers; legal professionals).

In Chapter 5, Dr. Robert Barkin, Dr. Kluft, and I summarize
the current state of knowledge regarding use of medication in
MPD patients. We point out that the MPD patient is subject to
the same side effects and adverse effects of any drug that the
general population is subject to and caution that the use of
psychoactive drugs is further complicated by the unpredictable
and often paradoxical responses seen in the MPD patient and
his or her alter personalities: Different personalities respond
differently to the same dose of the same drug. Only the drug
therapy that is absolutely required to treat the patient's entire
personality system should be used. Caution is advocated in
choosing drugs and dosage levels.

Dr. Cornelia Wilbur's discussion of psychoanalysis and MPD
in Chapter 6 makes it clear that the analyst should thoroughly
understand the etiological importance of dissociative capacity
and childhood experience of severe abuse. Dissociation is the
patient's principal defense, but the analyst is likely to encounter
any or all of the methods of ego defense described in the theoretical literature of psychoanalysis.

In Chapter 7, Dr. David Caul, Dr. Roberta Sachs, and I draw
on considerable experience with group psychotherapy of MPD
patients to elucidate this approach to treatment. Carefully selected and screened MPD patients can benefit from group psychotherapy that enhances and facilitates individual therapy.
Group therapy is always a complement to individual, never a
substitute. Used in conjunction with individual therapy, the
group experience provides an opportunity for characteristically
secretive, isolationist patients to learn interaction, acceptance,
tolerance, and other skills required for social functionability

and complements and stimulates their ongoing individual psychotherapy. Selection criteria for patients, recommendations for group setting and structure, therapeutic approach, and the importance of cotherapists are discussed.

Dr. Sachs, in Chapter 8, uses the 3-P model to structure the social support interventions that help maximize the effectiveness of psychotherapy. These include family interventions to stop abuse of a child or interrupt a family abuse cycle, marital therapy, parenting programs, incest groups to offer support to past victims, assertiveness training groups, peer networks, alcohol and drug abuse groups, and others.

In the final chapter of this book, Dr. Frank Putnam proposes a future direction for the advancement of the study of MPD. He proposes a multicenter collaborative study that could have both individual center and group components. This would be a good way to rapidly collect large numbers of patients and allow for standardized analysis of the data obtained from them and to encourage researchers nationwide to cooperate rather than compete. Such a study group had its first meeting at the Second International Conference on Multiple Personality/Dissociative States in 1985 and is looking into funding now.

Collectively, the nine chapters manifest the coalescence of clinical and research understanding of MPD into effective therapeutic approaches that provide great hope for future scientific advances.

An introduction to the first book on the treatment of MPD would not be complete without mentioning people who probably will never publish in this area but are key figures in furthering the therapy and study of dissociation. They are three people from Rush-Presbyterian-St. Luke's Medical Center who have contributed greatly to the field: Jan Fawcett, M.D., Chairman, Department of Psychiatry; Leo M. Henikoff, M.D., President; and Gary E. Kaatz, M.B.A., Associate Vice President/Associate Administrator, Medical Sciences & Services. Without their help, we would be neither so advanced nor making such rapid progress. Their support and encouragement have been responsible for obtaining the finances to establish the first and second International Conference on Multiple Personality/Dissociative States as well as an inpatient Psychiatric Trauma/Dissociative Disorders Unit currently being formed for treatment and research at Rush-Presbyterian-St. Luke's Medical Center.

It will provide treatment, training, and research for acute psychiatric trauma such as that suffered by rape victims, as well as the chronic psychiatric trauma seen in MPD, other dissociative disorders, and posttraumatic stress disorder.

Finally, I wish to express sincere gratitude to James Breeling, Muriel White, and Debbie Klenotic for their invaluable editorial assistance in the preparation of this book.

REFERENCES

American Psychiatric Association: Diagnostic and Statistical Manual of Mental Disorders (Third Edition). Washington, DC, American Psychiatric Association, 1980

Braun BG: Hypnosis for multiple personalities, in Clinical Hypnosis in Medicine. Edited by Wain HJ. Chicago, Year Book Medical Publishers, 1980

Braun BG: Psychophysiologic phenomena in multiple personality and hypnosis. Am J Clin Hypn 16:124–137, 1983

Braun BG: Foreword, in Symposium on Multiple Personality. Edited by Braun BG. Psychiatr Clin North Am 7:1–2, 1984a

Braun BG: Towards a theory of multiple personality and other dissociative phenomena, in Symposium on Multiple Personality. Edited by Braun BG. Psychiatr Clin North Am 7:171–193, 1984b

Braun BG: Dissociation: behavior, affect, sensation and knowledge, in Dissociative Disorders 1985: Proceedings of the Second International Conference on Multiple Personality/Dissociative States. Edited by Braun BG. Chicago, Rush University, 1985

Braun BG, Sachs RG: The development of multiple personality disorder: predisposing, precipitating and perpetuating factors, in Childhood Antecedents to Multiple Personality. Edited by Kluft RP. Washington, DC, American Psychiatric Press, 1985

Coons PM: The differential diagnosis of multiple personality disorder, in Symposium on Multiple Personality. Edited by Braun BG. Psychiatr Clin North Am 7:51–68, 1984

Kluft RP: Aspects of treatment of multiple personality disorder. Psychiatric Annals 14:51–56, 1984

Kluft RP: The natural history of multiple personality disorder, in Childhood Antecedents to Multiple Personality. Edited by Kluft RP. Washington, DC, American Psychiatric Press, 1985

Putnam FW, Post RM, Guroff JJ, et al: One hundred cases of multiple personality disorder (New Research Abstract No. 77). Presented at the annual meeting of the American Psychiatric Association, New York, 1983

Putnam FW, Guroff JJ, Silberman EK, et al: The clinical phenomenology of multiple personality disorder: 100 recent cases. J Clin Psychiatry 47:285–293, 1986

1

Issues in the Psychotherapy of Multiple Personality Disorder

Bennett G. Braun, M.D.

1

Issues in the Psychotherapy
of Multiple Personality Disorder

Multiple personality disorder (MPD) has been reclassified by the American Psychiatric Association (APA; 1980) in its *Diagnostic and Statistical Manual of Mental Disorders, Third Edition (DSM–III)* as one of four dissociative disorders. The essential feature of all such disorders is "a sudden, temporary alteration in the normally integrative functions of consciousness, identity, or motor behavior" (p. 253). The specific criteria that differentiate MPD from other dissociative disorders are 1) the existence within the individual of two or more distinct personalities, each dominant at different times; 2) the personality that is dominant at any particular time determines the individual's behavior; and 3) each individual personality is complex and integrated with its own unique behavior patterns and social relationships. In addition, I proffer that each of these criteria should be observed on more than one occasion (that is, there should be consistency over time) before the formal diagnosis of MPD is made (Braun 1985a).

The author wishes to acknowledge the editorial assistance of Edward J. Frischholz. Preparation of this chapter was partially funded by a grant from Mr. and Mrs. J. Mahoney.

Although diagnoses of MPD were frequent around the turn of the century, a dramatic decrease in the reported incidence of this disorder appeared after 1910. Rosenbaum (1980) speculated that Bleuler's introduction of the term *schizophrenia* around 1911 led to misdiagnosis of many MPD patients as schizophrenic. Indeed, in their recent study of 100 consecutive MPD cases, Putnam et al. (1983) reported that some were previously misdiagnosed as schizophrenic. Multiple personality disorder patients have been misdiagnosed as suffering from a variety of other psychiatric problems as well.

Another attempt to account for the post-1910 decline in the incidence of MPD is Larmore, Ludwig, and Cain's (1977) proposal that because MPD was identified most often through hypnosis, the disorder could be an artifact of hypnotic suggestion. If it were, it did not merit classification as a genuine diagnostic entity. However, it has been argued (Braun 1984b; Kluft 1982) that although MPD is not a by-product of hypnotic suggestion, some superficial symptoms of MPD can be elicited in highly hypnotizable subjects. Indeed, several investigators have observed that MPD patients tend to be significantly more hypnotizable than normal subjects or other clinical groups (Bliss 1983; Lipman, Braun, and Frischholz 1984). These findings suggest that tests of hypnotizability may be useful in the differential diagnosis of MPD.

In 1944 a review of the literature by Taylor and Martin found only 76 documented cases of MPD. However in the last decade the number of reported MPD cases has increased more than tenfold (Braun 1984c). This raises a new question: Why the dramatic increase in the incidence of MPD over the last decade?

One factor that has been associated with the increase in the number of reported MPD cases is a growing public awareness and popular fascination with this disorder. For example, the film *The Three Faces of Eve* and the books about Sybil and Billy Milligan are widely known. In addition, improved diagnostic criteria for MPD may have facilitated diagnostic precision. In contrast to its classification as one of the hysterical neuroses in DSM–II (APA 1968), its current classification (DSM–III; APA 1980) as a dissociative disorder is much more specific. The credibility of this explanation is supported by the finding of Putnam et al. (1983) that it takes an average of 6.8 years after first entry into the mental health system before the typical MPD patient is accurately diagnosed. I have observed a similar figure (6.88 years) in a study of 126 cases by different therapists (unpublished data, October 1985).

Although we are now beginning to be able to reliably identify MPD, we still do not clearly understand what causes and maintains the symptoms of this disorder. Unfortunately, most theories about MPD formed before 1944 were based on clinical observation of only a few cases or a single case study. However, during the last decade, a number of investigating practitioners have systematized their observations on a large number of MPD cases (Bliss 1980; Braun 1980, 1984c, 1985; Fagan and McMahon 1984; Kluft 1984a, 1984b; Putnam et al. 1983). Although most of these clinicians have not yet formulated a comprehensive theory about MPD, they have made some important observations about some of its distinguishing features.

Two recent theories about MPD have been useful in identifying the unique therapeutic needs of patients suffering from this disorder. The first of these is Kluft's (1984a) four-factor theory, which attempts to identify the various factors associated with the initiation and course of MPD. The other theory has been called the 3-P model of MPD (Braun and Sachs 1985) because it focuses on the predisposing, precipitating, and perpetuating factors that are associated with development of the syndrome. Because the 3-P model forms the basis for the 13 psychotherapeutic considerations I introduce later in this chapter, a brief description of the model is in order.

THE 3-P MODEL OF MPD

The 3-P model of MPD is diagrammed in Figure 1. Two predisposing factors are hypothesized to be necessary: 1) an inborn biological/psychological capacity to dissociate that is usually identified by excellent responsivity to hypnosis and 2) repeated exposure to an inconsistently stressful environment. The inconsistency is in the patient's receiving love and abuse for the same behavior, at unpredictable times. An abusive family environment has been the source of this inconsistent stress in the vast majority of MPD cases studied so far. However, other events such as the death of a family member, frequent geographic relocation, and cultural dislocation can also be identified as

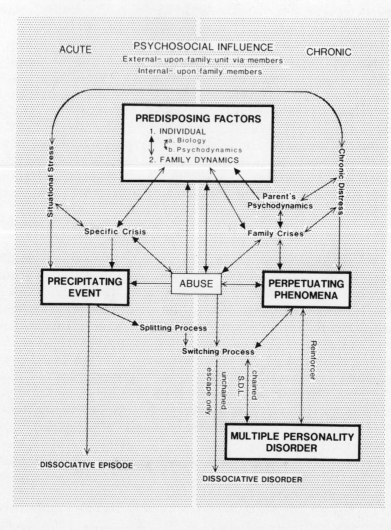

Figure 1. The 3-P model of multiple personality disorder.

sources of stress. Both of these predisposing factors are necessary for MPD to develop. Neither alone is sufficient.

The precipitating event in the 3-P model refers to a specific overwhelming traumatic episode to which the potential MPD patient responded by dissociating. If such events are not common in the environment of a patient with a dissociative capacity, then this typically results in a specific dissociative episode. Dissociative episodes are necessary but not sufficient conditions for the development of MPD. Many persons have a number of dissociative episodes throughout the course of their lives. As long as these episodes are not linked by a common affective theme and/or neurophysiological state (Braun 1984d), the person is unlikely to develop MPD.

The perpetuating phenomen associated with the development of MPD are interactive behaviors usually with the abuser and enabler and include separate memories that the patient ultimately links together by a common affective theme. For example, the child who has been abused starts to have pleasant and unpleasant memories of his or her parents. After continuous exposure to inconsistently abusive situations, the patient with dissociative capacity begins to file the memories of these traumatic events separately, and they begin to take on a life history of their own. For each fragment of affectively linked memories, a specific adaptive response to similar traumatic experiences develops. This chaining together of memories and development of associated response patterns is perpetuated by continuous unpredictable environmental trauma (Braun 1984d). Gradually the patient's personality is split because the different adaptive responses to the trauma have become functionally separated by an amnestic barrier. Thus, the patient is not aware that he or she is viewed by others as behaving inconsistently. This leads to the development of different personality states, each of which has its own adaptive function in the face of a particular kind of trauma.

DISSOCIATION AND MPD

To dissociate means "to sever the association of one thing from another" (Braun 1984d, p. 171). To this I would now add that what we see as MPD, especially in children, may well be a disorder of lack of association, since a significant association may never have been achieved from which to be dissociated. This makes developmental sense. When we speak of dissociation in the clinical context, we are usually referring to a defensive process. This is unfortunate because normal healthy individuals with a dissociative capacity do so even in the absence of psychological trauma (Frischholz 1985). For example, many people become so absorbed while watching a movie or a play that they temporarily lose awareness of where they are and find themselves strongly identifying with the actors in the drama (Hilgard 1970; Spiegel 1974; Tellegen and Atkinson 1974). However, these dissociative episodes are unlikely to become united by a common affective theme if they do not occur with sufficient frequency or if their occurrence can be predicted.

Highly traumatic events promote the use of dissociation as a psychological/behavioral defense in persons with an inborn biopsychological capacity to dissociate. If the dissociative individual's psychosocial environment is chronically and inconsistently permeated with traumatic events, then the individual instinctively resorts to dissociation as a defense because the trauma is simultaneously perceived as unpredictable and overwhelming. Such persons are likely to develop MPD especially if inconsistency of love and abuse is present and repeated. If the individual's psychosocial environment has a low potential for psychological trauma, then this person is less likely to use dissociation as a defense and typically is a normal, highly hypnotizable individual. However, in individuals with little or no dissociative capacity, the occurrence of chronic but unpredictable traumatic events is likely to stimulate denial as the primary psychological defense. Such individuals are likely to develop a psychiatric disorder other than MPD.

The trauma is usually associated with some form of inconsistent and unpredictable abuse. For example, a child may be severely beaten or affectionately hugged for the same behavior on different occasions. This usually begins at an early age in the family environment. When an individual with dissociative capacity uses it to defend against such abuse for the first time, he or she learns that the horrible memory can be kept out of conscious awareness. If the abuse is chronic and inconsistent, then dissociation becomes the preferred form of defense because it minimizes the perception of trauma.

IMPLICATIONS OF THE 3-P MODEL FOR TREATMENT

The 3-P model has many implications for treatment with MPD patients. Because its major assumption is that dissociation is used defensively as a fragmentation/compartmentalization process, the major thrust of psychotherapy clearly should be toward reassociating these fragmented thought processes into increasingly complex structures until full integration can be ultimately achieved. Another treatment consideration is based on the observation that MPD patients have a long history of being inconsistently abused by authority figures and in fact contribute to perpetuating this cycle of abuse. Therefore, the psychotherapist should make a marked effort to be both caring and consistent to the patient and to avoid the countertransference that will inevitably be stimulated by the patient's transferential projected reenactment in attempt to gain mastery.

On the basis of the 3-P model, 13 issues can be identified as basic considerations in the psychotherapy of MPD: 1) developing trust, 2) making and sharing the diagnosis, 3) communicating with each personality state, 4) contracting, 5) gathering history, 6) working with each personality state's problems, 7) undertaking special procedures, 8) developing interpersonality communication, 9) achieving resolution/integration, 10) developing new behaviors and coping skills, 11) networking and using social support systems, 12) solidifying gains, and 13) following up. This linear order is based on my own work with and observations of MPD patients and a need to create order. It is not a binding order; for most effective psychotherapy, issues may be interchanged or repeated. For example, issues of trust often have to be dealt with before each significant movement in the therapeutic process.

Developing Trust

The development of trust is important in treating any psychiatric disorder, but it is especially significant in the treatment of MPD. Complete mutual honesty is essential, and this can be accomplished only if both the therapist and the patient have the right to refuse to answer questions. Therefore, what is said can be counted upon without prejudice. In this regard, it is extremely important for the therapist to address four specific issues. First, the therapist must be consistent and yet flexible. Multiple personality disorder patients are used to dealing with inconsistent authority figures who are perceived as being both rigid and unpredictable. The therapist must know that the patient will attempt to manipulate him or her throughout the course of diagnosis and treatment and must not take it personally. The MPD patient will continuously try to set up the therapist so that he or she appears to be untrustworthy and unpredictable. In addition, the therapist must be able to set limits yet be prepared to stretch them at times when it would not make a major difference to the primary treatment or the ward staff.

Second, the therapist must not personalize any accusations made by the patient. This means that the therapist must do his or her best to be aware of countertransference and not become defensive. Multiple personality disorder patients will repeatedly test the therapist and his/her patience throughout the course of treatment. The therapist can expect this to happen and accept it as part of the patient's problem.

Third, MPD patients are masters of the double bind because this is the style of interaction and communication they experienced in their families of origin. They, like other victims of abuse, recreate situations for mastery. The therapist must be careful to avoid the MPD patient's use of the double bind. For example, if an MPD patient complains of lower abdominal pain, the physician must decide between two responses: 1) to ignore the patient's complaints or 2) to take the diagnostic and therapeutic action to relieve the patient's complaints. If the physician ignores the patient's complaints, then the patient can claim that the doctor does not pay attention to what he or she says. If the physician performs a routine abdominal, pelvic, and rectal examination, the patient can react with rage because the procedure is redolent of the abuse endured as a child. In either case, the physician is set up to appear neglectful or abusive. This situation is best handled by sticking with the facts, the medical needs, and good medical judgment. Then when the patient claims he or she was raped, the level of distortion can be made clear. We cannot protect our patients from the memories of their past abuses, and accepting guilt by association will only play into this maladaptive thought process and its distortions.

Fourth, the issue of trust will be called into question at each major point in therapy. The therapist must be careful not to react to this as an intentional affront. Multiple personality disorder patients have been abused in an inconsistent and unpredictable way. This partial reinforcement schedule for mistrust is very difficult to extinguish. Working on each major therapy issue is scary, and fear becomes the stimulus for the reactivation of mistrust.

Making and Sharing the Diagnosis

Making the diagnosis of MPD is not easy. The therapist must be careful to document consistency of the symptoms of MPD over several different occasions. Once the diagnosis is made, the therapist must share it with the patient. The timing of this revelation is a matter of therapeutic judgment. If the therapist shares the diagnosis with the patient before a trusting relationship has sufficiently developed, then the patient may get scared and leave treatment. If the therapist waits too long, then the patient may feel that he or she is not understood by the therapist and so leave treatment. When the interpretation is properly timed and accepted by the patient, the therapist can still expect some form of acting out to occur. Although nothing has actually changed, the secret has been exposed and this produces great fear. In addition, the therapist must be prepared for a cyclical pattern of accepting/rejecting the MPD diagnosis throughout the early and middle phases of treatment.

Communicating With Each Personality State

In communicating with each personality state, it is important that the therapist give credence to the information provided by each personality state. Typically, the therapist is overwhelmed by data. The novelty and quantity of data provided can make it difficult for the therapist to recognize different personalities. The therapist must let the patient know that he or she cannot remember every detail associated with each personality state. After the treatment has progressed and personalities begin to

merge, the therapist may again not recognize specific personalities because of other personalities that appear to be present
simultaneously with the host or alternate personality. One valuable way of communicating with each personality state is to use
hypnosis to facilitate the switching process, thus bringing it
under both the therapist's and the patient's control (Braun 1980,
1984a; Kluft 1982). This method is needed less and less frequently as therapy progresses, except for crises, resistances, and
certain procedures.

Contracting

Once the therapist has begun to collect data about each personality state, contracting with the patient to set limits becomes
essential to the progress of therapy. Four issues are relevant to
contracting. First, the therapist should make specific contracts
about the type and duration of treatment and/or the use of
special procedures. Second, the therapist should contract with
the whole personality system so that each personality state is
made responsible for what he or she individually says and does.
It is also useful to find one personality state who can speak for
the entire system. This forces the start of co-consciousness. When
doing this the therapist should note what is expressed not only
verbally but also nonverbally (including ideomotor signals). Third,
a contract is needed not to split off new personalities or fragments, or therapy will be endless. Fourth, and most important,
the therapist should make a specific contract that there is to be
no suicide or homicide. I approach this contract by asking the
patient to repeat the following phrase without necessarily meaning it and then asking how the patient would modify it so he
or she could live with it: "I will not hurt myself or kill myself,
nor anyone else external or internal, either accidentally or on
purpose at any time" (see Braun 1980, 1984a). The negotiable
points are the duration of the contract and the ability to hurt
others as protection from unprovoked external attack. If I cannot get a contract that is agreeable and binding, then hospitalization is a must. If one gets a time-limited contract, it must be
renegotiated prior to expiration or this will be perceived as an
implicit suggestion to act out. A modification of the time limit
might specify "one week or until we talk face to face, which

ever comes last." This covers the eventuality of an emergency or natural disaster interfering with the next scheduled visit.

Gathering History

The therapist begins to collect and organize data. History must be examined to learn five things about each personality or fragment: 1) who—the name or identifier of each personality state so that he or she can be easily addressed in the future; 2) when—the genesis of each personality state and the duration of time that it has executive control of the body; 3) why—why each personality state appeared, in terms of precipitating and perpetuating events associated with its development (this information might have to be obtained from another personality state) and why it is present at this time in life and/or treatment; 4) where—where the patient was at the time of this personality state's creation, where each personality state fits in the power structure, and where each personality fits into the system of personalities (see mapping below); and 5) what—the function of each personality state and how he or she aids the system as a whole. It is also interesting to learn from individual personality states exactly how each believes he or she was created. Care must be taken when obtaining this information; if the therapist becomes overinvested in its discovery, the progress of therapy may be retarded.

Working With Each Personality State's Problems

When history gathering has given the therapist an idea of the structure of the system, then work can begin on the individual problems of each personality state. This involves focusing on each personality state and sticking to the subject at hand. The therapist should generally not be too distracted by other personalities and new material competing for attention. Limits must be set regarding the amount of time to be spent with each personality state. Often because of time lost in switching, the different personalities feel slighted or believe that the therapist unilaterally reduced their treatment time.

It is not possible to deal with every problem or traumatic event experienced by every personality or fragment. Techniques must be developed to group the issues or to help one personality state be the therapist for others and do some of the therapy internally between sessions.

Another problem is dealing with somatic memories. This is the reexperiencing of specific traumatic memories along with their physiological concomitants. For example, the patient may remember being burned in the past and an actual blister may accompany this verbal report (Braun 1983b). Recall and reexperiencing of trauma is often perceived as if it were actually happening now.

When interacting with MPD patients, the therapist must work at several levels simultaneously. Having a quiet-room session using full leather restraints is not appropriate, nor is any abreactive technique, if a cognitive tree is not available on which to hang and integrate the emotions, behavior, and thought processes in order to make them congruent. Gathering emotions or facts is useless if they cannot be integrated. Abreaction, without cognitive structure, can be dangerous in an MPD patient because it can activate traumatic memories for which the patient has no defense or coping skill. This in turn can lead to an escalation of acting-out behavior and psychological or physical collapse.

Undertaking Special Procedures

Five special procedures can be used at specific times in therapy to uncover data and to help the patient's progress by developing mastery. These are 1) mapping, 2) sand worlds, 3) use of the quiet room and full leather restraints, 4) occupational therapy techniques, and 5) hypnosis. I developed the first three in conjunction with Dr. Roberta Sachs.

Mapping permits a more complex organization of the data that have been collected during the course of psychotherapy. The therapist, but preferably the patient, can draw or chart out the system(s) of personalities and their functions. As therapy progresses, the maps change and thus help to document the patient's progress over time. Maps provide ideas for the direction of therapy as well as how, among whom, and when to do integrations (Braun and Sachs 1986).

Sand worlds are constructed by the patient at appropriate times in therapy and are worked with individually as well as analyzed sequentially over time. These are created using a standard-sized shallow box filled with sand in which all types of small figures and toys are placed to express what the patient is thinking and feeling. Certain objects will take on special significance. This is a form of "play therapy" for these adult patients that allows them, child personalities, and fragments that are nonverbal or preverbal to communicate. It also assists verbal communication. Corrective experiences can be suggested or obtained. Secrets can also be expressed and understood in this manner without having to "tell" (Sachs and Braun 1986).

In the hospital, one might want to judiciously use the quiet room and/or full leather restraints as an adjunct to a special therapeutic procedure. This will produce safety for the patient and the staff, thereby facilitating the expression of emotion in a planned, controlled, and safe manner (Braun and Sachs 1985b; Young 1985).

Special occupational therapy techniques such as using and/ or throwing clay, building things, or participating in art therapy have been especially useful in helping the patient express feelings and the therapist understand the patient's "secrets."

Hypnosis is often thought to be a special technique, but it is merely a tool to be used in conjunction with whatever type of therapy is being effectively used. It is safer and easier than drug-assisted interviews, which also have been used successfully (Braun 1980, 1984a; Horevitz 1983; Kluft 1982, 1983, 1984a, 1985).

Developing Interpersonality Communication

The therapist should encourage interpersonality communication as an early step to co-consciousness and integration. This promotes the sharing of knowledge and information about various experiences in the patient's developmental history, which in turn promotes fusion as different personality states learn about the specific adaptive functions each has in protecting the system. It also allows for a sharing of needs and desires so that mutual influence and co-consciousness can be obtained. Interpersonality-state communication can be done at first via the therapist, then more directly via internal group therapy (Caul 1984). Traditional group therapy for MPD has been described by others (see Coons and Bradley [1985] and Chapter 7 in this book).

Achieving Resolution/Integration

To achieve resolution of the patient's problems and integration of his or her personalities, the therapist must deal with power struggles among the different personality states over who will remain. Some personality states may fear they will die if they become integrated. This issue must be addressed directly. The different personalities need to be reassured that they all will contribute to the remaining whole. Often this can explained using the analogy of mixing red and white paint to get a larger volume of pink paint. Both colors contribute to the final product, which has a larger volume (i.e., is more functional) than either color originally.

An acceptable but less stable form of resolution is a co-consciousness or a mutual cooperation that is less than complete integration. Some patients choose to stop therapy at this point. Although I believe this result has a significntly less chance for long-term stability, I must respect the patient's wish to not face certain issues, in the hope that he or she will return when help is needed. I always work for full integration.

The specific psychotherapeutic techniques for integration depend on the therapist's imagination and what is significant for the patient. Often, hypnosis is useful at this point.

At one time, the terms *integration* and *fusion* were used interchangeably to mean the same thing. Currently, however, *integration* means the process by which thought and physiological processes are mixed and solidified. *Fusion* is defined as the bringing together of separate personalities. Integration starts before fusion and continues after it.

Integration/fusion does not have to be effected in the hospital, but at times it is necessary. It can occur spontaneously, but often a ritual is found to be useful by the patient. The ritual should be tailored to the patient's needs and the personalities involved to be meaningful. This may be facilitated by hypnosis. Good fusions that become lasting integrations are accompanied by physiological changes (Braun 1983a, 1983b, 1984a). After fusion, the patient needs time to heal. He or she will often report changes in vision, hearing, and other sensations as well as periods of confusion. These will normalize over time (usually completely by three months).

Developing New Behaviors and Coping Skills

The therapist needs now to help the patient develop new behaviors and coping skills. This involves learning and practice in a safe environment to enable new responses to become integrated into a response system. At this point, patients often recognize their conflicting thought patterns and this can be quite upsetting for them. They need reassurance that this is a normal problem that will resolve with time and experience. Multiple personality disorder patients have particular trouble dealing with ambiguity because they are accustomed to switching to a personality state congruent with a particular event or thought process. Patients must be taught to deal with ambivalence, to accept having two or more feelings at one time, and to weigh their decisions before acting on them. They must learn new ways of dealing with life rather than running away via dissociation.

At this point in therapy, many MPD patients feel as if they are less able to function effectively and that they are losing their creativity. While it is true that patients may have more trouble making decisions and dealing with ambivalences, this clears as thinking solidifies.

Networking and Using Social Support Systems

Networking and social support groups are useful psychotherapeutic adjuncts. Because the MPD patient has so much information to integrate, his or her needs can seem overwhelming and exhausting to a single therapist. Social support systems are especially effective in this regard because they return the patient to the community and help prevent therapist burnout.

The major advantage to using existing social support groups is that they provide a safe environment for the patient to learn and behaviorally rehearse skills that do not ordinarily come up in psychotherapy. For example, vocational counselors can help the MPD patient learn new job communication skills and market existing job skills effectively. Various tutorial groups can help MPD patients learn job skills that they missed while dissociating in school or during job training. Groups such as Alcoholics Anonymous, Alanon, and Parents Anonymous as well as the patient's family can be quite useful in therapy (see Chapter 8).

Sometimes a marital or family intervention can be a useful adjunct to the main treatment approach by helping the MPD patient to deal immediately with his or her primary social relationships (Kluft et al. 1984). Parenting groups can help the MPD parent learn effective parenting skills and mitigate the likelihood of further child abuse.

Solidifying Gains

Solidifying gains is a continuation and polishing of new behaviors and coping skills. Such practice, with its associated successes and failures, allows for smooth chaining of thought processes so they will become more automatic. At this point many MPD patients who complained of experiencing slowed thinking after integration find that their normal pace of thinking has returned.

Following Up

After integration has been achieved, follow-up visits are recommended to ensure that integration is maintained. The importance of follow-up in helping a former MPD patient to stay healthy is emphasized by Kluft (1984a, 1985, Chapter 2 in this book). During follow-up visits, the therapist can use hypnosis to detect the existence of additional personality states. If some are found, treatment can be reinitiated. If the integration comes apart because of stress, it can be repaired in a small fraction of the time that therapy took originally.

These 13 therapeutic issues are broadly applicable in the treatment of dissociative disorders in which the therapist may encounter multiple personalities or personality fragments. Figure 2 postulates that dissociation may be conceptualized as a continuum from nonpathological dissociation (normal) through dissociative disorders including amnesias, fugue states, and depersonalization to atypical dissociative disorder and the various forms of MPD.

In atypical dissociative disorder with features of multiple personality, the therapist may encounter personality fragments that must be identified, understood, and eventually incorporated into a whole personality. This patient is one who dissociates

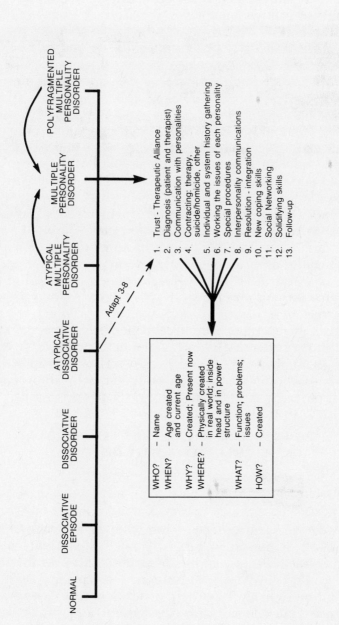

Figure 2. Continuum of dissociation and a treatment approach for multiple personality disorder and its variants.

frequently for various periods of time, but the dissociative episodes linked and shaped by intermittent life experiences do not qualify as full personalities.

In atypical MPD, the patient initially may not appear to have multiple personalities at all. There is little or no disruption in knowledge between the personalities because they exchange factual information but not the affective component of memory among themselves, for example, while the patient is asleep; thus, even though behavior, affect, and sensation are dissociated, the retention of continuous knowledge among the personalities may be erroneously perceived by the therapist as full memory. Under sufficient stress, the atypical MPD patient will decompensate and present as a typical MPD patient (Braun 1985b).

Treatment of the patient with polyfragmented MPD should seek first to coalesce the personality fragments around issues of time, age, trauma, or life events in order to form a cluster of personalities that can be integrated and treated as the personality of a typical MPD. The fragments encountered in this patient may exhibit a range from short to continuous life histories, affect, and behavior.

Kluft has also operationalized treatment outcome criteria (Kluft 1984a), and reported both short- and long-term follow-up data on a large number of MPD cases (Kluft 1984a, Chapter 2 in this book). Collectively, these data suggest that the prognosis for psychotherapy and healing of MPD patients is good.

OTHER SALIENT ISSUES IN THE TREATMENT OF MULTIPLE PERSONALITY DISORDER

The Need to Hospitalize

Whether to hospitalize depends on whether the patient may hurt himself or herself or others. If such a possibility seems likely, then the MPD patient should be hospitalized as any other patient would be. (A word of caution: Dissociation may make acting out more likely, because individual personalities do not experience ambivalence, only the system as a whole does. Therefore, a switch will upset the power dynamic.) Hospitalization may also be necessary to deal with potential decompensation, rage reactions, or a severe inability to function or to undertake special therapeutic procedures with safety.

A safe hospital may be the only way to help a patient face, recall, and express memories of severe emotional and physical traumas. In many of the patients, the rage is so severe that they not only dissociate to escape from it but use dissociation to protect their therapist and society from their acting out when the denial or dissociative barrier breaks down. Some information, for example forced participation since childhood in satanistic cult worship entailing ritualistic sex, human sacrifice, and cannibalism is so terrifying and overwhelming that it requires the assistance of a trained staff available 24 hours a day to help these patients cope. Dr. Roberta Sachs and I have successfully aided nine patients from different parts of the United States who had experienced such terrifying circumstances, and I know of at least 50 others.

Though this represents the extreme end of the continuum, many of the tortures inflicted on other MPD patients as children were just as overwhelming. In addition to the various overwhelming abuses, many MPD patients have been threatened with their lives if they tell anyone about what they have been subjected to and/or observed. Therefore, they keep the secret and are unable to process their experiences, as are many victims of trauma, which results in posttraumatic stress disorder (PTSD).

The association among MPD, dissociation, and PTSD has been discussed (Putnam 1984; Spiegel 1984). One could consider PTSD a dissociative disorder that includes dissociation via both intrusion (intrusive thoughts, nightmares, and hypervigilance) and denial (inattention, amnesia, and constriction of thought processes), as suggested by Horowitz (1976). In this light it also makes sense to look at MPD as a special case of chronic PTSD. This viewpoint promotes a blending of thought on medication and psychotherapeutic strategies that will improve our understanding of how to treat these complex clinical syndromes (Braun 1986).

Because MPD patients are generally reluctant or afraid to talk about their experiences, expressive therapies such as occupational, art, music, and movement therapy and also psychodrama are quite useful in allowing the patient to express conflict and even specific information without "telling." Once this is done, the information can be worked with and integrated into more traditional psychotherapy. Care must be taken to pace the disclosure of the information so that patient and/or staff are not overwhelmed by the amount and type of disclosures. This is especially true of psychodrama.

Given the severity of the abuse, the risk of violence, the reluctance to disclose, and the loss of memories to consciousness, the length of hospital stay becomes an area of concern, especially in this era of cost cutting. Not all hospitalizations of MPD patients need to be lengthy. Hospitalizations of my patients have ranged from three days to 15 months.

At the ultra-short end of hospital stay, 3 to 10 days, comes the special procedures and quiet-room sessions. These hospitalizations are specifically designed for a predetermined issue that has been preworked on an outpatient basis, except for the procedure. A short hospitalization may be indicated for an integration that requires protection and rest.

In the short zone, 2 to 4 weeks, there is diagnostic evaluation and treatment planning or some medication evaluation and adjustment. The 2- to 8-week range presents more difficult diagnostic problems, most notably those with extreme trust or violence issues.

The mid-range of 8 to 12 weeks is rare. This is because when one exceeds an eight-week stay there will often be significant regression. Effectively dealing with this regression generally requires 12 to 16 weeks of hospitalization.

Patients that require stays of six months or longer usually have a mixture of symptoms presenting as severe suicidal/homicidal ideation, severe issues of trust, inability to care for themselves, and/or other severe concomitant psychopathology, such as an overall borderline presentation, severe depression, or polyfragmentation. Also these patients may have significant concurrent medical problems.

Patients with violent suicidal/homicidal outbreaks or ideation are the hardest to predict in terms of length of stay. They may recompensate in a few weeks or may require intensive psychotherapy with medication to help them restructure enough to be safe. One must be able to observe safety, contracts, and behavior for a sufficient period of time to be comfortable with the issue of safety, since MPD patients may switch personalities and thereby lose control of thoughts and behavior.

Some areas of concern in treating MPD patients, especially

in the hospital, are 1) splitting, 2) limit setting, and 3) the establishment of boundaries.

Splitting. Splitting can occur in all imaginable combinations and at several levels simultaneously. These levels can be physician and colleagues, physician and staff, staff and staff, staff and other patients, other patients with each other, and all imaginable combinations even including administration and staff from other uninvolved units. Preventing this requires a great deal of open communication and information processing so a proper milieu can be maintained. Good nursing support and coordination is even more essential with MPD patients than with borderline patients.

Limit Setting. Setting behavioral limits is essential not only to preserve the therapist's sanity but also to control therapy and allow it to proceed. Multiple personality patients test and retest in all conceivable ways. Limits need to range from rigid to firm to flexible and must always be observed. There are four levels of limits: 1) those that must never be exceeded for to do so would irreparably damage the therapeutic alliance (e.g., a serious attack on the therapist or his or her family), 2) those that are very important (e.g., escaping from the hospital, suicide attempts, child abuse), 3) those that give the therapist firm control of medication and the therapy process but allow for varying amounts of patient input, and 4) those that are negotiable (e.g., bed time, length of passes, short-term therapy goals, and some of the ramifications if contracts are broken).

Establishment of Boundaries. Boundaries must be established and maintained (Duda et al. 1985). These include personal boundaries such as privacy of the therapist and confidentiality for the patient.

Physical touch is also a personal boundary. Touch is an essential and potent therapeutic tool and as such must be treated with great respect. I will not touch a patient without prior permission from the particular personality that is out and without a reason for the touch. This reason must include a hypothesis as to the patient's response. By doing so, if an unusual or unexpected response occurs, I will recognize it and better respond. Unplanned touching, even out of caring, can have painful con-

sequences such as the patient's misperceiving it as pain or seduction. There may be an opposite-sex personality present in
the body, or a homosexual or lesbian personality. Behavior
resembling sexual seduction must be guarded against. Because
more than 80 percent of these patients have been sexually abused
(Putnam 1983). Sexual abuse is a major frame of reference for
their perception of and interaction with the world.

Another major boundary that must be observed is time. Multiple personality disorder patients, because of their many facets,
are also seductive at the intellectual level. They have a pressure
to get everything done yesterday, which is a major trap. The
therapy must be paced. The therapist must control the rate and
amount of material revealed. Extended sessions should be
planned in advance, and crises must be minimized by dealing
only with the crisis issue and resisting the temptation to do
further exploration or therapy even though the patient is ripe
for it.

Medication

Judicious use of medication can be of great value during crises.
It can give the therapist enough leverage to help the psychotherapy be effective in restoring order. However, the use of
medication with MPD patients can also be problematic for several reasons. First, different personality states have been observed to have different responses to, as well as different
tolerances of, the same amount of a given drug. Second, the
potential for unconscious overmedication is always present. For
example, one personality may take a medication without being
aware that another personality has already taken a similar dose.
Third, the use of antipsychotic medications may further impair
the MPD patient's reality testing skills and promote further
switching and splitting. In this case, the long-term use of antipsychotic medications may have no therapeutic effect and may
even be perpetuating some of the symptoms of this syndrome.
However, a single dose of antipsychotic medication is sometimes
useful during a crisis to help reestablish control.

The psychotherapist who attempts to treat MPD should be
aware of hospitalization and medication issues. Space does not
permit further elaboration here. Interested readers are referred to other sources for a more detailed discussion of these

topics (see Chapter 5 in this book; Braun and Sachs 1985b; Kluft 1984b; Putnam 1984).

CONCLUSIONS

The recent increase in the incidence of MPD has promoted a more careful and extensive study of this disorder. Both the four-factor theory of Kluft (1982) and the 3-P model that Dr. Sachs and I (1985a) developed provide a clinically useful theoretical framework for planning the course of psychotherapy. Few specific interventions have been recommended for resolving the various treatment issues identified in the present discussion because little empirical data exist to support the superiority of one psychotherapeutic orientation over another. Therefore, how the psychotherapist resolves these issues depends on his or her own creativity and the patient's responsiveness.

REFERENCES

American Psychiatric Association: Diagnostic and Statistical Manual of Mental Disorders (Third Edition). Washington, DC, American Psychiatric Association, 1980

Bliss EL: Multiple personalities. Arch Gen Psychiatry 37:1388–1397, 1980

Bliss EL: Multiple personality, related disorders, and hypnosis. Am J Clin Hypn 26:114–123, 1983

Braun BG: Hypnosis for multiple personalities, in Clinical Hypnosis in Medicine. Edited by Wain HJ. Chicago, Year Book Publishers, 1980

Braun BG: Neurophysiologic changes in multiple pesonality due to integration: a preliminary report. Am Clin Hypn 26:84–92, 1983a

Braun BG: Psychophysiologic phenomena in multiple personality and hypnosis. Am J Clin Hypn 26:124–137, 1983b

Braun BG: Uses of hypnosis with multiple personality. Psychiatric Annals 14:34–40, 1984a

Braun BG: Hypnosis creates multiple personality: myth or reality? Int J Clin Exp Hypn 32:191–197, 1984b

Braun BG: [Foreword.] Symposium on Multiple Personality. Edited by Braun BG. Psychiatr Clin North Am 7:1–2, 1984c

Braun BG: Towards a theory of multiple personality and other dissociative phenomena, in Symposium on Multiple Personality. Edited by Braun BG. Psychiatr Clin North Am 7:171–194, 1984d

Braun BG: The transgenerational incidence of dissociation and multiple personality disorder, in Childhood Antecedents of Multiple Personality. Edited by Kluft RP. Washington, DC, American Psychiatric Press, 1985a

Braun BG: Dissociation: behavior, affect, sensation, knowledge, in Dissociative Disorders 1985: Proceedings of the Second International Conference on Multiple Personality/Dissociative States. Edited by Braun BG. Chicago, Rush University, 1985b

Braun BG: Dissociation: an overview. Presented at the annual meeting of the American Psychiatric Association, Washington, DC, 1986

Braun BG, Sachs RG: The development of multiple personality disorder: predisposing, precipitating, and perpetuating factors, in Childhood Antecedents of Multiple Personality. Edited by Kluft RP. Washington, DC, American Psychiatric Press, 1985a

Braun BG, Sachs RG: Creation of an inpatient program for dissociative disorders, in Dissociative Disorders 1985: Proceedings of the Second International Conference on Multiple Personality/Dissociative States. Edited by Braun BG. Chicago, Rush University, 1985b

Braun BG, Sachs RG: The structure of the MPD's system of personalities, in Dissociative Disorders 1986: Proceedings of the Third International Conference on Multiple Personality/Dissociative States. Edited by Braun BG. Chicago, Rush University, 1986

Caul D: Group and videotape techniques for multiple personality disorder. Psychiatric Annals 14:43–50, 1984

Coons PM, Bradley K: Group psychotherapy with multiple personality patients. J Nerv Ment Dis 173:515–521, 1985

Duda D, Caninga C, Geary RN: Nursing care of the hospitalized multiple personality disorder patient: a developmental process, in Dissociative Disorders 1985: Proceedings of the Second International Conference on Multiple Personality/Dissociative States. Edited by Braun BG. Chicago, Rush University, 1985

Fagan J, McMahon PP: Incipient multiple personality in childhood: four cases. J Nerv Ment Dis 172:26–36, 1984

Frischholz EJ: The relationship among dissociation, hypnosis, and child abuse in the development of multiple personality disorder, in Childhood Antecedents of Multiple Personality. Edited by Kluft RP. Washington, DC, American Psychiatric Press, 1985

Hilgard J: Personality and Hypnosis. Chicago, University of Chicago Press, 1970

Horevitz RP: Hypnosis for multiple personality disorder: a framework for beginning. Am J Clin Hypn 28:138–145, 1983

Horowitz MJ: Stress Response Syndromes. New York, Jason Aronson, 1976

Kluft RP: Etiology of multiple personality. Presented at the annual meeting of the American Psychiatric Association, New Orleans, May 1981

Kluft RP: Varieties of hypnotic interventions in the treatment of multiple personality. Am J Clin Hypn 24:230–240, 1982

Kluft RP: Hypnotherapeutic crisis intervention in multiple personality. Am J Clin Hypn 28:73–83, 1983

Kluft RP: Treatment of multiple personality disorder: a study of 33 cases, in Symposium on Multiple Personality. Edited by Braun BG. Psychiatr Clin North Am 7:9–29, 1984a

Kluft RP: Multiple personality in childhood, in Symposium on Multiple Personality. Edited by Braun BG. Psychiatr Clin North Am 7:121–134, 1984b

Kluft RP: The treatment of multiple personality disorder: current concepts. Directions in Psychiatry (Volume 5). Edited by Flach FF. New York, Hatherleigh, 1985a

Kluft RP, Sachs RG: Multiple personality. Int J Fam Ther 5:283–302, 1984

Larmore K, Ludwig A, Cain R: Multiple personality: an objective case study. Br J Psychiatry 131:35–40, 1977

Lipman LS, Braun BG, Frischholz EJ: Hypnotizability and multiple personality disorder, in Dissociative Disorders 1984: Proceedings of the First International Conference on Multiple Personality/Dissociative States. Edited by Braun BG. Chicago, Rush University, 1984

Putnam FW, Post RM, Guroff JJ, et al: One hundred cases of multiple personality disorder (New Research Abstract No. 77). Presented at the annual meeting of the American Psychiatric Association, New York, 1983

Putnam FW: The psychophysiologic investigation of multiple personality disorder, in Symposium on Multiple Personality. Edited by Braun BG. Psychiatr Clin North Am 7:31–40, 1984

Rosenbaum M: The role of the term schizophrenia in the decline of diagnoses of multiple personality. Arch Gen Psychiatry 37:1383–1385, 1980

Sachs RG, Braun BG: The use of sand worlds with the MPD patient, in Dissociative Disorders 1986: Proceedings of the Third International Conference on Multiple Personality/Dissociative States. Edited by Braun BG. Chicago, Rush University, 1986

Spiegel D: Multiple personality as a post-traumatic stress disorder, in Symposium on Multiple Personality. Edited by Braun BG. Psychiatr Clin North Am 7:101–110, 1984

Spiegel H: The grade V syndrome. Int J Clin Exp Hypn 22:303–319, 1974

Taylor WS, Martin MF: Multiple personality. Journal of Abnormal Social Psycholology 39:281–300, 1944

Tellegen A, Atkinson G: Openness to absorbing and self-altering experiences ("absorption"), a trait related to hypnotic susceptibility. J Abnorm Psychol 83:268–277, 1974

Young WC: What to do 'till the friendly one comes, in Dissociative Disorders 1985: Proceedings of the Second International Conference on Multiple Personality/Dissociative States. Edited by Braun BG. Chicago, Rush University, 1985

2

Personality Unification in Multiple Personality Disorder: A Follow-Up Study

Richard P. Kluft, M.D.

2

Personality Unification in Multiple Personality Disorder: A Follow-Up Study

Multiple personality disorder (MPD) is a severe chronic dissociative disorder characterized by a disturbance of memory and identity (Nemiah 1985). Putnam et al. (1984) observed that "the existence of multiple amnestic episodes, together with the presence of alternating separate and distinct identities, distinguishes multiple personality disorder from all other psychiatric syndromes" (p. 172). Until recently, this condition was considered a rarity. Its authenticity and its importance as a clinical syndrome were questioned. Many practitioners and researchers found and continue to find it difficult to view MPD with objective dispassion. The very nature of its manifest phenomena, which is often dramatic and flamboyant, seems to elicit both countertransferential fascination and countertransferential skepticism.

Similarly, the treatment of MPD is a controversial area of study. Although the first successful treatment of MPD was described as far back as 1840 (Ellenberger 1970), the alleged rarity of the disorder and the strongly polarized reactions that have surrounded it throughout its history have, until recently, weighed against MPD's becoming the subject of serious scientific inquiry. Multiple personality disorder was still regarded as a rare entity in 1944, when Taylor and Martin indicated that only approximately 100 cases had been reported and that some were questionable. They reviewed 76 of the 100 cases. Clearly, since publication of the *Diagnostic and Statistical Manual of Mental Disorders (Third Edition) (DSM–III*; American Psychiatric Association 1980), it is difficult for clinicians of today to retrospectively assess reports from an era in which medical science could not reliably distinguish individuals afflicted by luetic, epileptic, schizophrenic, affective, schizoaffective, borderline, or posttraumatic stress pathologies from persons suffering from a dissociative disorder. Moreover, the evaluation of reports from a time before investigators became sophisticated about the impact of their suggestions and inquiries on the phenomena they observed is problematic.

Since 1944, however, and most dramatically since 1974, when the first mention of a large series of MPD patients seen by a contemporary clinician entered the literature (Allison 1974), there has been a rising tide of interest in this condition. By 1980, the literature contained more than 200 cases (Bliss 1980). Since then, large series of MPD patients have been noted by Beahrs (1982), Bliss (1980, 1984), Braun (1980, 1985), Clary et al. (1984), Coons (1985), Greaves (1980), Horevitz and Braun (1984), Kluft (1982, 1984c), Putnam et al. (1983), Schultz et al. (1985), and Solomon and Solomon (1982). Cohorts have ranged from 12 to more than 300 patients.

The reasons for this abrupt rise in the recognition and reporting of MPD cases are varied and have occasioned complex debate. Certainly media and lay attention to the celebrated cases of "Eve," "Sybil," and Billy Milligan brought MPD to the attention of professional audiences. It is hard to cite a major American television series that has not exploited the dramatic potential of MPD. The reclassification of MPD in *DSM–III* as a freestanding entity among the dissociative disorders also brought this condition to the attention of mental health professionals (American Psychiatric Association 1980). Many have become aware of the compelling parallels and similarities between MPD and posttraumatic stress disorder (Spiegel 1984). Excitement has been generated by neuropsychophysiological research findings (Braun 1983; Brende 1984; Coons et al. 1982; Putnam et al. 1982; Putnam 1984a, 1984b) that suggest that the study of MPD may offer insights into psychosomatics and brain function and also may constitute a paradigm for the exploration of the structures and processes of the human mind (Putnam 1984a, 1984b). Increased awareness of the prevalence of child abuse and incest has heightened clinicians' sensitivities to MPD, which is commonly the sequel to an abusive and/or overwhelming childhood (Putnam et al. 1983; Kluft 1984c; Wilbur 1984). In two studies comprising 100 and 309 cases each, 97 percent of the cases involved childhood mistreatment (Putnam et al. 1983; Schultz et al. 1985). Furthermore, the increasing awareness by women of issues related to gender has intensified concern about a condition that not only is related to abuse and exploitation but also is reported to have a four-to-one (Kluft 1984a) to nine-to-one (Greaves 1980) predominance of women among its victims. Finally, among the helping professions, a small group of dedicated teachers and clinicians have gradually raised consciousness about MPD.

However, the growing accord that MPD has long been seriously underdiagnosed and misdiagnosed is far from a consensus. Victor (1974) wondered if the diagnosis and treatment of MPD can constitute a folie à deux. Kline expressed concern whether patients with severe ego fragmentation are being erroneously labeled as having MPD (1984). Thigpen and Cleckley cautioned that patients may try to "achieve" the diagnosis and seek out therapists who will "sanction" it (1984). Orne, in Goleman (1985), warned against the diagnosis's being suggested by therapists. Spanos et al. (1985) suggested the condition would become manifest when the contextual inducements called for such enactment.

Many authors' misgivings are heightened when hypnosis enters the diagnostic and therapeutic processes. In recent independent studies, Braun (1984b) and Kluft (1982) explored the literature on hypnosis and MPD to see if the former appeared to lead to the latter. It did not. Kluft also replicated several hypnotic procedures that had been described as creating MPD (1985d). Two observations summarize a middle-ground view of the subject: Gruenewald (1984), who reviewed these issues from both the clinical and the theoretical perspective, commented, "Although injudicious use of hypnosis may have a variety of untoward effects, causation *de novo* of multiple personality does not seem to be one of them" (p. 175); Kluft (1982) observed, "Phenomena analogous to and bearing dramatic but superficial resemblance to clinical multiple personality can be elicited experimentally or in a clinical situation if one tries to do so or makes technical errors . . . phenomena can be elicited by hypnosis and overinterpreted as multiple personality" (p. 232).

Debate over the true prevalence of MPD and the reasons for its sudden emergence as a not uncommon contemporary clinical syndrome is likely to continue into the foreseeable future, but in the meantime psychiatrists must be prepared to encounter such patients and undertake their treatment. Throughout the history of medicine, suffering individuals have presented themselves for help long before their conditions could be understood definitively and comprehensively by those who try to alleviate their discomfort and ameliorate their distress.

When today's psychiatrist attempts to learn about the treatment of MPD, he or she will find both articles that advocate and articles that countermand or question virtually every major therapeutic approach (Kluft 1985a). Close inspection of a number of articles in which certain treatment principles are illustrated and/or advocated reveals that the authors either do not specify their data base or offer their advice on the basis of experience with a single case that did not enjoy a successful outcome. In this chapter I describe a follow-up study involving a number of MPD patients ($N = 52$) who were treated to the point of fusion and sequentially reassessed. The general treatment approach used was psychodynamic psychotherapy facilitated by hypnosis (Kluft 1982, 1984c). This approach is consistent with a treatment plan described by Braun (1980; see also Chapter 1 in this book), it follows most of the guidelines suggested by Bowers et al. (1971), and its nonhypnotic aspects generally are similar to a treatment described by Wilbur (1984).

LITERATURE REVIEW

The growing literature on MPD was catalogued by Boor and Coons (1983). A number of the authors described psychoanalytic approaches to MPD (Lasky 1978; Marmer 1980; Lampl-De Groot 1981). Multiple personality disorder patients whose personalities are accessible and cooperative without hypnosis and are otherwise analyzable may profit from analysis, but cases are known in which one personality was analyzed and others were never discovered (Kluft 1985a). The behavioral literature is sparse (Caddy 1985; Kohlenberg 1973; Price and Hess 1979). In a recent unpublished presentation (Association for the Advancement of Behavioral Therapy 1984), Drs. Klonoff and Janata described an elegant behavioral paradigm. The authors found that they could suppress the overt manifestations of MPD but that in the absence of abreaction and working through, their patients relapsed readily. Pending reports of several successful treatments with adequate follow-up, the behavioral treatment of MPD must be regarded as experimental (Kluft 1985a). Braun argues in Chapter 1 that abreaction requires a preexisting cognitive structure adequate for understanding and interpreting the abreacted experience if lasting effect is to occur. This is similar to emotional congruency's being required if behavioral change is to be lasting.

A number of authors in the literature catalogued by Boor and Coons described family intervention approaches to treating MPD: Davis and Osherson (1977), Beal (1978), Levenson and Berry (1983), and Kluft et al. (1984). Family therapy has not proved to be a viable primary treatment modality, but it may have excellent ancillary uses. Its use with a traumatizing family of origin is associated with a high incidence of crises, but it may be quite helpful to other genuinely concerned persons in the patient's life space and thus may be of great support to the patient.

The syndrome generally has not proved to be responsive to medication but may coexist with other conditions that are drug responsive (see Chapter 5). Patients may manifest target symptoms that require palliative treatment (Kluft 1984b). The use of videotaped Amytal interviews was described by Hall et al. (1978), and the use of videotaped hypnotic sessions was described by Caul (1984). Caul also described the creation of an internal group therapy among the personalities (1984). Multiple personality disorder patients have not proved to be good candidates for inclusion in heterogeneous group therapies unless they share a common bond with the others in a group, for example, being an incest survivor. Homogeneous groups of MPD patients are difficult to control but can be a valuable ancillary tool (Coons and Bradley 1985; see also Chapters 7 and 8 in this book). Such patients may do well in structured occupational art, movement, and music therapy groups used as adjuncts to inpatient treatments (Kluft 1984b).

Abundant literature is available on the use of hypnosis in treating MPD; in recent studies applicable techniques were catalogued (Braun 1980, 1984c; Kluft 1982). Fears that hypnosis can create or worsen MPD prevail, but several recent reviews have shown that such concerns are highly overstated (Braun 1984b; Gruenewald 1984; Kluft 1982; Sutcliffe and Jones 1962). Unpublished research by Braun and Sachs indicates that the collaboration of several therapists using several modalities can be productive.

At this point in time, the majority of successful treatments of MPD have been accomplished by clinicians who provide supportive psychodynamic psychotherapy that is facilitated when necessary by hypnotic interventions. Bowers et al. (1971) and Wilbur (1984) described such approaches.

BACKGROUND OF THE PRESENT STUDY

When I began working with MPD patients, I was uncertain whether integration of the separate personalities was generally feasible or desirable. I took the empirical stance that if I attended to the overall treatment of each individual suffering with MPD, this issue would be resolved by clinical experience. Using supportive–expressive psychoanalytic psychotherapy with occasional hypnosis to access alters, retrieve data, and support integration, I found that patients whose personalities worked toward cooperation and integration fared better than did those whose personalities tried to cooperate but zealously guarded their separateness. In fact, personalities who gave cooperation high priority in spite of their avowed wish to stay separate found themselves integrating and/or ultimately asked me to help them integrate. These experiences caused me to surmise that replacing dividedness with unity was a practical and desirable rather than a theoretically optimal goal. I also learned that the appearance of unity could be misleading. If it were achieved via the suppression, extrusion, banishment, or alleged departure of other entities, the patient remained depleted, and relapse into dividedness was nearly universal (Kluft 1982). This led me to abandon approaches that failed to accept all personalities as valuable parts of an overall whole.

Once it became clear that unification was associated with superior clinical results and therefore was a desirable outcome, I began to study apparent unifications over time to assess their stability. In performing sequential reassessments of ostensibly fused patients over extended periods of time, I found a great deal of relapse phenomena and began to wonder if stable integration were possible. When I scrutinized the circumstances of the relapses, however, I found that most of them were related to the incompleteness of the antecedent treatment interventions and difficulties in the therapeutic alliances within those treatments. My findings in no way suggested that stable integration is impossible.

I found six categories of problems that contributed to relapse. Often several coexisted in a given relapse. First, some personalities had pretended to be gone or had refused to emerge and later either confessed they had evaded detection to avoid being confronted with painful memories and issues or made this clear by subsequent verbalizations and behaviors. This could be understood as a variety of flight into health, a common event in the psychotherapy of all conditions. The unusual features of MPD often make this type of event difficult to detect. Furthermore, once a patient has faced a massive amount of traumatic material, it is difficult to suspect that he or she is feigning health in order to avoid facing even more traumata of a still more upsetting nature.

Second, many personalities secretly persisted to exist throughout therapy, in some cases playing along with therapy, to preserve their narcissistic investments in separateness. Some of these personalities simply wished to survive, albeit covertly. Others planned to take over as soon as therapy came to an end. Still others took the stance that therapy had been decided upon by some for the sake of all and there was no real reason for them to change in any way. In essence, there had never been a true therapeutic alliance among these personalities.

Constituting a third category of situations that contributed to relapse, some personalities had felt that they had to remain available to the otherwise unified individual, who, they felt, could not be safe without their assistance and protection. They usually became quite cooperative once discovered, although they often were tenacious about retaining separateness for long periods of time before integrating. In essence, these personalities had doubted the safety of the proposed outcome of therapy and rather than truly invest themselves in a process of fusion, had held back and retained a "wait and see" attitude.

The fourth type of problem that contributed to relapse was that the personalities' reasons for being had not received adequate working through. They still held even more traumatic memories and/or needed to do further abreactive or interpretive work in their areas of concern. Again, it was quite difficult for both therapist and patient to realize, having gone through what seemed to be an arduous and intensive processing of difficult material, that they had only done a fraction of the work that would ultimately prove necessary to achieve a definitive outcome.

A fifth contributor to relapse in MPD cases was that to the extent that fusion had been emphasized during treatment, the message had been conveyed that a prompt fusion would be gratifying to the therapist. This caused some patients to feel impelled to feign fusion and/or not report evidence of further dividedness in order to please the therapist. Pressing for rapid fusion proved to be counterproductive.

The sixth and final problem that I found contributed to relapse was that many patients had perceived fusion as a threat, for a variety of reasons. They had often felt they could not be open about their fears lest the therapist be upset or lest discussion of the fears lead to their being talked into fusion before they were ready. Hence, they had held back.

Attending to these six types of difficulties and deemphasizing fusion greatly speeded fusion and reduced relapse rates. The patients felt their anxieties were better appreciated and more fully addressed. A slower pace of treatment yielded more rapid and stable results.

In studying the epidemiology of relapses, I defined a relapse as the return of personalities to separate entities or the emergence of new or previously undiscovered personalities. Although the latter two events are not true relapses, I classified them as such to 1) avoid inadvertent overstatement of positive results and 2) anticipate the criticism that such events are iatrogenic and/or factitious and might reflect the patients' perception that they were being encouraged to display or would benefit from displaying such phenomena once again.

I found that the relapse occurrences clustered into three time

Table 1. The Epidemiology of Relapses in Multiple Personality Disorder

Time	Usual Causes
Up to 1 week	Fusion unwelcome—coerced or done to please or evade Insufficient working through Rerepression
Up to 3 months	Analogous issues to those of fused alters under discussion Unsuspected related alters Characterological issues Some layering Rerepression
Up to 27 months	Layering Object loss or threat of it Death of abuser Terminal illness Rerepression Egosyntonic autohypnotic regression Withheld data Characterological issues

zones after apparent achievement of fusion (see Table 1). Within each of these time zones, a different group of causes seemed prevalent.

Patients who experienced relapse shortly after apparent integration generally did so for reasons different from those of patients who experienced relapse weeks, months, or years later. The early or first group consisted of patients whose integrations were friable and showed signs of coming undone very rapidly, that is, within a week. When a fusion occurred in the face of great external pressure, took place in spite of marked inner opposition by some personalities, was experienced as coercive, or took place in the presence of any of the aforementioned six types of problems, the prognosis for rapid return to dividedness verged on 100 percent.

Causes of relapses that occurred during the second time zone, from one week to three months after apparent fusion, differed from those of relapses that occurred in the first time zone. Many times, a number of personalities had some common connection to a particular set of experiences and/or issues. Therefore if therapy had focused on an issue that touched several personalities, the apparent fusing of one personality into the developing whole sometimes triggered work on the same area by another personality. This led to reemergence of the ostensibly fused personality and/or the flushing to the surface of previously unknown personalities with similar concerns. (The latter possibility is one form of the "layering" phenomenon [Kluft 1984c]). Work with all related issues and personalities may be necessary to pave the way for lasting integrations. Some patients tried to rerepress painful data and redissociate; some tried to undo fusions. Also, at this point, patients whose nondissociative coping skills were poor, having passed through a brief honeymoon phase, found themselves overwhelmed by ongoing and new stressors. Lacking other ways of dealing effectively with their distress and dysphoria, they were readily drawn toward the reestablishment of a dissociative mode of defense.

Relapses that occurred within the third time zone, after three months of apparent fusion, were due to some of the aforementioned six contributors to relapse, as well as other factors. Layering was the most common cause of relapse in the third time zone, followed by intercurrent life events, such as the illness or loss of loved ones, the death of an abuser (which often seemed to facilitate further rerepression, of still more traumata, and the unearthing of previously well-hidden personalities), or the onset of a terminal illness. (Although this did not occur in any of the patients whose relapses I'm describing in this chapter, my experience with other patients who did not 27 months of fusion documents that catastrophic events, such as rape, can precipitate relapse any time after fusion in a certain percentage of MPD patients.) Among this group of patients, I found those who tried to reestablish their MPD by autohypnosis and those who withheld crucial information, thereby leaving important conflicts unresolved and leaving themselves vulnerable to a return to reliance on dissociative defenses.

What happens in a relapse caused by layering is that as the initially encountered personalities of an MPD patient are treated and their issues worked through, other groups or layers of personalities, who had no apparent or acknowledged presence in the course of the treatment up to that point, are now encountered.

Sometimes these layers consist of active personalities who simply had been unknown to the personalities involved in therapy. Sometimes the layers consist of personalities who had been masked by the activities and manifestations of the known personalities. In other situations, the newly discovered personalities are ones who had been suppressed by known personalities, and when the known personalities became fused, the suppression ceased. Some layers consist of personalities who had been dormant for years or who had been evading therapy quite willfully.

In any case, as the therapy proceeds, layered personalities may be triggered, enabled, or forced to emerge. Sometimes emergence appears related to these personalities' contiguity to the issues of the personalities who fused last. Sometimes a personality, now fused, had in some way camouflaged the existence of others. On other occasions the reassembling of memories and understandings from the accounts that had been offered by several now-fused personalities allowed the discovery of others.

As an example, in an obese patient several personalities had claimed responsibility for her compulsive overeating. However, the thorough exploration of their dynamics and their integration was not followed by any improvement. The personality into whom they had integrated seemed genuinely unaware of the persistent gorging. No known personality could be related to the eating behaviors. A few weeks later, the therapist encountered a cluster of several previously unknown personalities who overate ferociously. They confessed that they had exerted their impact through the personalities who had recently been integrated. When despite these newly discovered personalities' contracting against it, the overeating continued, the therapist used hypnosis to search for and find yet another layer of personalities related to the overeating. Work with and integration of all these layers ended the overeating. In another case, the integration of several personalities reduced the patient's internal confusion to the point that he realized he could not account for two years of his life. Inquiry led to the discovery of two previously unknown personalities who had dominated behavior during the missing period.

The discovery of layering within a week of apparent complete integration is unusual; thereafter it becomes more common. Beginning three months after apparent integration, its incidence is rather steady for approximately two years. Because relapse in general becomes less common with the passage of time and other early relapse forms decline in incidence, layering becomes the most common cause of relapse long after fusion. In over 100 cases I have studied thus far (including those not described here), 90 percent of layering relapses occurred within 27 months of apparent fusion. The remaining 10 percent were encountered over a period of several years.

My sequential study of patients after apparent self-described fusion revealed that certain findings were characteristic of patients who remained integrated at least three months. Because these findings rarely characterized cases of patients who relapsed rapidly, they could be made operational as a clinically derived definition of fusion. Thus fusion can be defined as three stable months of 1) continuity of contemporary memory, 2) absence of overt behavioral signs of multiplicity, 3) subjective sense of unity, 4) the absence of alternate personalities upon hypnotic reexploration (unless the patient was psychoanalyzed), 5) transference modifications consistent with the bringing together of personalities, and 6) clinical evidence that the unified patient's self-representation included acknowledgments of attitudes and awarenesses that were previously segregated in separate personalities (Kluft 1982). Sixty percent of patients who achieved these criteria showed no signs of dissociation on all successive reevaluations. In other cases, the personalities who reemerged were not as fully defined in reemergence as they had been before, and usually fused rapidly. One-third of the relapses thereafter were clearly triggered by life stresses and one-third by the emergence of previously unknown personalities (layering). In another third, there were reprises of prior and/or short-lived new alters, usually accompanied by layering. As a result, it seemed prudent to regard an integration of less than 3 months as an apparent fusion, an integration of 3 months or more a fusion, and one of 27 months or more a stable fusion. I conducted a study to explore the stability of integration in MPD patients considered to have achieved a stable fusion.

In the present study, the terms *fusion* and *integration* were understood as synonyms. Recently there has been a tendency to define fusion as a point in time at which a particular entity ceases to be separate and/or the entire individual achieves unity. Integration has been defined as an ongoing process of undoing all aspects of dissociative dividedness, a process that begins be-

fore any alters yield their separateness and continues after personalities have joined into one. This study was begun before
the distinction was widely discussed; furthermore, it is difficult
to use this definition of integration for research purposes.

METHOD

I had acquired a large series of MPD patients referred for
treatment or discovered during case-finding research. From
among 106 MPD patients who fulfilled fusion criteria for three
months or more, 52 who fulfilled the additional criteria for
stable fusion were selected for further study. Only three fell
short of *DSM–III* criteria for MPD (American Psychiatric Association 1980) and the amnesia and repeated observation of
spontaneous dissociative phenomena that are additional criteria
advocated by Coons (1980, 1984, 1985) and Braun (1985), respectively. Data on 33 of these subjects are reported elsewhere
(Kluft 1984c). The subjects included 14 males (26.9 percent)
and 38 females (73.1 percent). Fifty subjects were white, one
was black, and one was oriental. They ranged from 8 to 69 years
of age at diagnosis; their mental health careers prior to the
diagnosis of MPD ranged from nil to more than 30 years. Three
had concomitant bipolar disorders. Most had some borderline
features, but a formal *DSM–III* diagnosis of borderline personality disorder could be made only for nine (17.3 percent).

The majority of patients were referred with the MPD diagnosis already made or suspected. Some were found during my
attempts to develop diagnostic protocols for the detection of
MPD (Kluft 1982, 1985b, 1985c, unpublished data). I saw all
the patients in a private setting. All reassessment procedures
were undertaken either in ongoing postfusion therapy or in
the course of following up on patients who had agreed to return
for periodic evaluations after termination.

All patients in this series were treated by me. Those I saw in
consultation or in the process of supervising other therapists
were not readily available for sequential assessment. If a patient
was already in treatment prior to the diagnosis of MPD, that
treatment format was continued unless it was proving unsuccessful. For example, one patient dissociated while in the fourth
year of a supervised classical psychoanalysis. Because all personalities agreed to remain in analysis and made progress, this

treatment was continued to a successful resolution. Another patient was diagnosed when she dissociated during a behavioral exposure regimen. This treatment format allowed her personality to be brought to the surface and to deal with traumatic events but did not lead to integration. Integration was effected with a single hypnotic intervention and endured throughout an extensive follow-up period.

Generally, the treatments were psychoanalytic in conceptualization, supportive–expressive in stance, and eclectic in technique. Patients were followed in a problem-oriented fashion, and treatment decisions were often made on an informal decision-theory model, using both the patient as his or her own control and data amassed from other MPD patients. The modal patient was seen once or twice weekly, up to daily when in crisis, and was given prolonged sessions to deal with difficult and painful material for which profound abreaction was anticipated. Twenty-three patients (44.2 percent) had been hospitalized during their treatment for MPD. Fifty-one (98.1 percent) had at least one hypnotherapeutic intervention, not including hypnotic screening for the stability of integration during postfusion follow-up. Approximately four out of five had at least one personality that integrated during a hypnotherapeutic procedure.

Treatment was characterized by efforts to draw all the personalities into the therapy, according them equal respect, and paying diligent attention to the therapeutic alliance. When personalities could be accessed without hypnosis or the personality in control could and would report the others' productions, perceived as inner auditory hallucinations, the treatment resembled a basic but rather active and supportive psychoanalytic psychotherapy with interpretations occasionally directed to more than one personality. When this was difficult to achieve, hypnosis was used to facilitate treatment. Usually, but not inevitably, after access to personalities was achieved by hypnosis on one or more occasions, the same access was possible later without hypnosis.

All patients understood that treatment would continue to the resolution of their overall difficulties and would not end at integration. The motivations for such socialization were twofold: 1) Early results showed that patients who interrupted treatment at the point of apparent fusion almost invariably relapsed, and 2) many patients feared that the therapist would end treatment upon integration and consequently evaded working toward that objective. The socialization spoke to these concerns. Furthermore, as termination neared, patients were asked if they would participate in follow-up assessments.

Patients undergoing sequential reassessment were evaluated between 27 months and 99 months after achieving integration. Assessment followed a nine-step protocol (for description, see Kluft 1985d) that, in brief, entails 1) conducting a clinical interview; 2) administering the Center for the Study of Dissociative States diagnostic schedule for MPD in its current version (Kluft, unpublished data); 3) inquiring in detail about the signs and symptoms that characterized the patient's previous manifestations of MPD; 4) obtaining a detailed interim chronology; 5) eliciting the patient's report of other people's expressed perceptions of the patient's apparent unity or residual dividedness; 6) exploring the patient's own perceptions of his or her unity or dividedness; 7) inquiring about all personalities without the use of hypnosis, attempting to summon those previously encountered during treatment, checking for the presence of layering (Kluft 1984c), and attempting to see if any new personalities have formed; 8) inquiring about personalities and so forth with hypnosis; and, when possible, 9) obtaining data from ancillary sources. Such a protocol may require portions of one to four 45-minute sessions to administer. The inquiry process was benign and generally well tolerated, even when the findings were disappointing to the patients (Kluft 1984c, 1985d).

Certain characteristics of these patients and the dissociative nature of their pathology often frustrate conventional interviewing methods. These include the patients' repression and denial, their fear of discovering and having to face still further dividedness and painful material, their wish to please the therapist by representing their treatments as successful, certain personalities' having remained without reportable behavioral evidences, and some personalities' evading discovery. For these reasons, the hypnotic inquiry often was the most productive element of the protocol in detecting subtle relapse events.

RESULTS

To avoid the inadvertent overstatement of gains, I registered any evidence of patient's use of dissociative defenses or manifestation of dividedness as a relapse event, regardless of whether it constituted a relapse in the sense of the return of symptoms believed to have been already identified and treated successfully. Therefore, the designation of relapse was not restricted to the discovery that a personality or personalities believed to have integrated had persisted or returned. It also was applied to the discovery of personalities who had not been detected in the course of the preintegration therapy and had never entered treatment and to instances in which a completely new personality had been formed. In a similar spirit, phenomena that fell short of diagnosable *DSM–III* MPD were enumerated as relapse phenomena as were those that had the more classic MPD manifestations. This latter decision was supported by recent findings that many patients who are diagnosed as classic cases of MPD have spent much of their lives not manifesting the condition in a florid and easily recognized manner (Kluft 1985c). Although perhaps 20 percent of MPD patients show the signs of MPD longitudinally over time, 80 percent manifest the signs only intermittently, and therefore provide only "windows of diagnosability" for classic MPD (Kluft 1985b).

Other considerations in these decisions included the skeptical stances that 1) newly discovered personalities—perhaps the overall phenomenology of MPD—were iatrogenically inspired and created and 2) the discovery of additional dividedness, and perhaps all purported manifestations of dividedness, could be understood as a factitious disorder motivated by the wish to hold and retain the therapist's attention. From either skeptical stance, the discovery of additional MPD phenomena would be perceived as a recurrence of the same epiphenomena of the initial therapeutic misadventure rather than as a further unfolding of a complex dissociative structure or the patient's new usage of a transiently abandoned defensive operation.

The 52 patients in the present study included 33 described in an earlier publication (Kluft 1984c) and the 19 therein noted who had achieved integration but either had not sustained it long enough to satisfy criteria for stable integration at that point in time or had not yet been thoroughly reassessed. Both groups are among the 106 integrated patients that I am attempting to follow longitudinally in an ongoing study. Together they represent those patients from the overall group that successfully have achieved integration by stated criteria (Kluft 1982), have maintained the appearance of fusion for a minimum of 27 months, and have been systematically reassessed thereafter. In order to facilitate comparison of the present with the earlier findings, both are provided in Table 2, the first of three summary tables.

Fifty-one of the 52 patients alleged a better quality of life and global improvement at the time of the reassessment. One man had been diagnosed as having multiple sclerosis a month before his reassessment and thus was quite distraught. Two patients who alleged improvement proved to have misrepresented themselves. One had feigned fusion and in fact was miserable (see Case 1). The second had retreated into a world of autohypnotic fantasy, and her statements could not be accorded face value. However, for 94.2 percent of the cohort, there was clear evidence of improved function and progress in life.

Only 11 patients (21.2 percent) were found to have had relapse events. Of these, only three (5.8 percent) had diagnosable *DSM–III* MPD. The only full relapse case among these three was the patient who had never really integrated. In another, who had 33 personalities, only one of those who had become part of a unified individual had again reseparated and was present (see Case 2). In the third, who had had five known personalities, two of these were separate again but were less well defined than they had been before their short-lived integrations. Also, two previously undiscovered personalities were found.

In sum, 94.2 percent had not relapsed into behaviorally manifest MPD, and of that 78.8 percent had not suffered residual or recurrent dissociative difficulties. These outcome findings are consistent with and nearly identical to the results reported for the first 33 of these patients, reported separately (Kluft 1984c). They suggest that when offered appropriate treatment and energetic follow-up, MPD patients can achieve a stable remission of the symptoms that characterize the condition and can live stable and productive lives as unified individuals.

These data also suggest that a certain percentage of MPD patients remain vulnerable to relapse and that follow-up is advisable. They also indicate aggressive reassessment is useful and should include hypnotic inquiry. Of the 11 patients who experienced relapse, only two were both able and willing to characterize their ongoing difficulties. The others were unaware,

Table 2. Summary Data

Number	Average age at fusion	Months therapy from diagnosis to fusion*	Number of personalities	Borderline organization	Full relapse	Full personality	Relapse Events		
							Returned personality	New personality	Layering
52 (33)	37.1 (36.1)	21.6 (21.6)	15.4 (13.9)	9 (5)	1 (1)	3 (2)	6 (6)	2 (2)	5 (3)

Note. Data in parentheses are from Kluft (1984c) study.
*The point of apparent fusion that proved lasting.

were denying, were withholding, or were just beginning to suspect they had a problem of some sort. The vigorous recheck protocol was without significant adverse impact (Kluft 1985d).

Certain trends noted previously (Kluft 1984c, 1985d) persisted in this larger cohort. Individuals with fewer personalities generally required shorter periods of treatment and were less prone to relapse (Table 3). Male patients tended to have fewer personalities, shorter treatments, and fewer relapses (Table 4). Relapse events were more common in individuals with greater numbers of personalities. In both the present study and the Kluft (1984c) study, 75 percent of the relapse events occurred in patients who had 18 or more personalities. In that group, the prevalence of relapse events was 0.6 events per patient; that is, 60 percent had relapse events. In patients with 17 or fewer personalities, approximately 8 percent had relapse events. Beyond these generalizations, no correlation seems to exist between relapse events and still greater degrees of complexity, although there are mild suggestions that increasing complexity usually but not invariably is correlated with longer periods of treatment prior to the achievement of integration. In this respect, the length of treatment of the patient with 110 personalities is misleading. Her 38 months of therapy involved more than twice as many sessions per week than did the therapy of the patients who had 86 and 88 personalities, respectively. Of the nine patients with strong borderline features, three experienced relapse events. Although such individuals are harder to treat to a point of stable fusion, they can achieve and sustain this goal.

Case examples of relapse events can familiarize the reader with MPD relapse presentations.

Case 1

A medical professional was very symptomatic and dysphoric but tried to maintain that all was well. She exerted herself to present a normal veneer to me and was more or less successful in this deception. I saw that she was minimizing her discomfort but did not discern either the full extent of her troubles or her ongoing dividedness. She denied all signs and symptoms on the reassessment protocol until I began the hypnotic inquiry. At that point, she broke trance and confessed she had feigned

Table 3. Relationships Among the Number of Personalities, Duration of Treatment, and Relapse Events

Duration and relapse	Number of personalities/number of patients									
	2/6	3/6	4/1	5/13	6/2	7/1	8/4	9/1	12/1	16/2
Average duration of treatment (months)*	6.5	5.2	24	10.4	31	30	21	30	18	34
Number of relapse events	0	0	0	0	1	1	1	0	0	0
	18/2	20/1	22/2	25/2	28/1	33/3	36/1	86/1	88/1	110/1
Average duration of treatment (months)*	27	60	36	36	36	28	24	42	48	38
Number of relapse events	2	1	0	1	1	3	0	0	0	1

Note. N = 52.
*The point of apparent fusion that proved lasting.

Table 4. Comparing Male and Female Patients

	Number	Percentage	Age at fusion (years)	Months of treatment*	Number of personalities	Percentage who experienced relapse events
Males	14	26.9	37.6	16.3	8.1	7.1
Females	38	73.1	37.6	23.1	18.0	26.3
Total	52	100.0	37.6	21.6	15.4	21.2

*The point of apparent fusion that proved lasting.

fusion and prematurely left treatment against my advice in the hope that she could avoid detection and resume her career. After several months of apparent success, she had become dysfunctional. All 18 previously known personalities were present, as were 14 others who had evaded detection. She repeated this pattern of feigned fusion at a later date, but this deception was rapidly detected.

Case 2

A woman with 33 alternate personalities, all integrated into one, had concluded a successful treatment. A year later, she learned that her husband had terminal lung cancer. After not working in 30 years, she suddenly had to support her family. She also had to care for her husband, on whom she had depended. A helper personality redissociated and was present at her reassessment interview with me. This helper personality set up a small business and then reintegrated. On subsequent reassessments over the course of years, this helper personality could not be found.

Case 3

A woman's unjust humiliation at work triggered her recovering, via dreams and transference fantasies, memories of profound humiliation at the hands of her father during traumata she had not remembered in her prior therapy. She was reassessed and found to have a reprise of a few of her previous personalities, who were no longer well defined and who did not assume executive control unless elicited by hypnosis. She also had a layer of personalities related to the newly discovered materials. The personalities said they could emerge but agreed that they would not do so outside of sessions because they felt assured of help in therapy. The patient's father did not deny that the newly recovered incidents had occurred. The memories were worked through and the personalities all integrated within months. The patient has been stable on subsequent rechecks over a 36-month period.

Case 4

A patient who had been integrated for three years showed signs of forgetfulness and was reassessed. Six protector personalities were found to have remained separate to see if fusion would work. Having decided that life as a unified individual was desirable, each personality was taking over incompletely for brief periods of time and then integrating slowly. Complete integration followed uneventfully.

Clearly, most of the relapse events fell far short of a recurrence of classic MPD and responded readily to treatment. Only two of the 11 patients who experienced relapse events remain dissociated in any manner as of this writing.

In another study, I reassessed patients who have had at least 63 months of apparent integration, that is, they have shown no dissociative residua for at least five years after satisfying fusion criteria. This indicates that long-term stability is feasible. However, one of these 13, after eight years of stability, suffered a two-week reprise of fragmentation and dissociation when she returned home unexpectedly early, entered her bedroom, and found her husband performing fellatio on another man. The personalities that formed were vague and fragmentary and appeared to be trying to augment an abortive attempt to repress what she had seen. When she accepted her circumstances, they ceased to be apparent or accessible. She has shown no dissociative residua in the 30 months since that event.

A second patient had been incapacitated for two decades prior to the diagnosis and treatment of his MPD. Achieving integration, he returned to the work force and was steadily employed for six years. He reported brief periods of time loss following a promotion and noted that when he recovered awareness, he found that work he had feared facing was lying completed on his desk. He was found to have an executive personality who had run his own small business more than 20 years earlier but had been inactive since then. Not encountered during therapy, this personality apparently had been triggered to reemerge after the promotion, when the patient was quite anxious about assuming leadership abilities.

DISCUSSION

These findings offer an encouraging prognosis for MPD. However, as for any data that are drawn from a single practice, it is presented without validation from other observers and is offered without controls of any sort. Hence, interpretations and inferences must be made with caution. Also, the results obtainable by an experienced practitioner working in a setting in which follow-up is ensured to all patients are unlikely to be replicated by a neophyte or a person unable to provide such ongoing continuity of care and the security it implies. Only ten (19.2 percent) of the present patients are now in any ongoing contact with me beyond periodic reassessment. These patients are still in phases of postfusion therapy, which sometimes is lengthier than the treatment required to achieve integration. It is hoped that this study will stimulate other investigators to not only institute their own follow-up studies but also to arrange for persons other than themselves to confirm the initial diagnosis and perform the sequential reassessments. It would be desirable to study the fate of MPD patients in treated, untreated, pseudotreated, and treatment without attention to MPD cohorts, but the data already amassed suggest that untreated patients do not recover spontaneously (Kluft 1985c), whereas treated patients fare well (Kluft 1984c). This information, the length of the treatment, and the fact that treatment refusers are a questionable control group, make it unlikely that such a study can be undertaken without logistic and ethical difficulties.

At this point in time, it appears that MPD has a good prognosis when intense treatment and continuity of care are available and patients are motivated to make use of it. The treatment is likely to be prolonged and difficult, and most patients will prove to have many more personalities than they initially appeared to have. The instability of gains until all personalities are identified and all issues and memories worked through and resolved has led to the appearance of gains being difficult to attain and transient at best. Actually, the failure of an integration is no more than an indicator that there is more work to be done. Because MPD patients' defenses are geared toward denial, disavowal, avoidance, and evasion of painful stimuli, treatments that end after the achievement of apparent unity and/ or fail to probe for ongoing problem areas are associated with a high probability of relapse events.

These results and those of a prior study (Kluft 1984c) suggest that certain factors are associated with more rapid treatment results and more favorable prognoses. However, all such factors must be weighed with caution, because the very fact that the patients in this study group were successfully treated may mean that they are atypical. For example, in this study, male patients appeared to be less complex, to recover more rapidly, and to relapse less readily. However, clinical experience indicates that more males than females decline or evade treatment, and this may bias the inferences one may draw from the present male MPD treatment cohort. Among adults, age differences do not appear to be a factor in prognosis for fusion. Youngsters with MPD integrate very rapidly compared with most adult patients (Kluft 1984d). Complexity appears to augur for a prolonged treatment and a greater likelihood of relapse events, but only up to a certain point. Very complex patients can attain and sustain integration. It appears that patients with 18 or more personalities have a harder time giving up dissociative defenses and are more likely to uncover sequential layers of additional personalities.

Concomitant diagnoses were not a focus of the present study. Unpublished data (Kluft) indicates that patients' areas of problematic ego strength and their degree of masochism, the personalities' narcissistic investments in separateness, patients' reinforcement from significant others to be multiple, and the presence of severe Axis Two pathology all complicate treatment, as does the presence of an extensive inner world of personalities who interact with one another in relationships of great complexity and/or intensity. When patients' current external life circumstances are difficult and/or patients remain enmeshed with their abusers, their treatment becomes singularly difficult because they rarely can tolerate the discontinuing of their dividedness and dissociative defenses. The coexistence of a drug-responsive affective disorder does not worsen prognosis, but when the affective disorder is difficult to control, treatment of the dissociative disorder per se is impaired.

SUMMARY

Results from this study of 52 MPD patients reassessed sequentially after their attaining integration suggest that the condition has an excellent prognosis if intense long-term psychotherapy is made available and the patients are motivated to pursue it.

REFERENCES

Allison RB: A new treatment approach for multiple personality. Am J Clin Hypn 17:15–32, 1974

American Psychiatric Association: Diagnostic and Statistical Manual of Mental Disorders (Third Edition). Washington, DC, American Psychiatric Association, 1980

Beahrs JO: Unity and Multiplicity. New York, Brunner/Mazel, 1982

Beal EW: The use of the extended family in the treatment of multiple personality. Am J Psychiatry 135:539–542, 1978

Bliss EL: Multiple personalities. Arch Gen Psychiatry 37:1388–1397, 1980

Bliss EL: Spontaneous self-hypnosis in multiple personality disorder, in Symposium on Multiple Personality. Edited by Braun BG. Psychiatr Clin North Am 7:135–148, 1984

Boor M, Coons PM: A comprehensive bibliography of literature pertaining to multiple personality. Psychol Rep 53:295–310, 1983

Bowers MK, Brecher-Marer S, Newton BW, et al: Therapy of multiple personality. Int J Clin Exp Hypn 19:57–65, 1971

Braun BG: Hypnosis for multiple personalities, in Clinical Hypnosis in Medicine. Edited by Wain HJ. Chicago, Year Book Publishers, 1980

Braun BG: Neurophysiological changes in multiple personality due to integration: a preliminary report. Am J Clin Hypn 26:84–92, 1983

Braun BG: [Foreword], in Symposium on Multiple Personality. Edited by Braun BG. Psychiatr Clin North Am 7:1–2, 1984a

Braun BG: Hypnosis creates multiple personality: Myth or reality? Int J Clin Exp Hypn 32:191–197, 1984b

Braun BG: Uses of hypnosis with multiple personality. Psychiatric Annals 14:34–40, 1984c

Braun BG: The transgenerational incidence of dissociation and multiple personality disorder: a preliminary report, in Childhood

Antecedents of Multiple Personality. Edited by Kluft RP. Washington, DC, American Psychiatric Press, 1985

Brende JO: The psychophysiological manifestations of dissociation: electrodermal responses in a multiple personality patient, in Symposium on Multiple Personality. Edited by Braun BG. Psychiatr Clin North Am 7:41–50, 1984

Caddy CR: Cognitive behavior therapy in the treatment of multiple personality. Behav Modif 9:267–292, 1985

Caul D: Group and videotape techniques for multiple personality disorder. Psychiatric Annals 14:43–50, 1984

Clary WF, Burstin, KJ, Carpenter JS: Multiple personality and borderline personality, in Symposium on Multiple Personality. Edited by Braun BG. Psychiatr Clin North Am 7:89–100, 1984

Cleigh Z: The three faces of Ruth. San Diego Tribune, April 18, 1985, E-1, E-10

Coons PM: Multiple personality: diagnostic considerations. J Clin Psychiatry 41:330–336, 1980

Coons PM: The differential diagnosis of multiple personality, in Symposium on Multiple Personality. Edited by Braun BG. Psychiatr Clin North Am 7:51–68, 1984

Coons PM: Children of parents with multiple personality disorder, in Childhood Antecedents of Multiple Personality Disorder. Edited by Kluft RP. Washington, DC, American Psychiatric Press, 1985

Coons PM, Bradley K: Group psychotherapy with multiple personality disorder patients. J Nerv Ment Dis 173:515–521, 1985

Coons PM, Milstein V, Marley C: EEG studies of two multiple personalities and a control. Arch Gen Psychiatry 39:823–825, 1982

Davis DH: Osherson A: The concurrent treatment of a multiple personality woman and her son. Am J Psychother 31:504–515, 1977

Ellenberger HF: The Discovery of the Unconscious. New York, Basic Books, 1970

Goleman D: New focus on multiple personality. New York Times, May 21, 1985, C1, C6

Greaves GB: Multiple personality: 165 years after Mary Reynolds. J Nerv Ment Dis 168:577–596, 1980

Gruenewald D: On the nature of multiple personality: comparisons with hypnosis. Int J Clin Exp Hypn 32:170–190, 1984

Hall RC, Le Cann AF, Schoolar JC: Amobarbital treatment of multiple personality. J Nerv Ment Dis 166:666–670, 1978

Horevitz RP, Braun BG: Are multiple personalities borderline? in

Symposium on Multiple Personality. Edited by Braun BG. Psychiatr Clin North Am 7:69–87, 1984

Kline MV: Multiple personality: facts and artifacts in relation to hypnotherapy. Int J Clin Exp Hypn 32:198–209, 1984

Kluft RP: Varieties of hypnotic interventions in the treatment of multiple personality. Am J Clin Hypn 24:230–240, 1982

Kluft RP: An introduction to multiple personality disorder. Psychiatric Annals 14:19–24, 1984a

Kluft RP: Aspects of the treatment of multiple personality disorder. Psychiatric Annals 14:51–55, 1984b

Kluft RP: Treatment of multiple personality disorder: a study of 33 cases, in Symposium on Multiple Personality. Edited by Braun BG. Psychiatr Clin North Am 7:9–29, 1984c

Kluft RP: Multiple personality in childhood, in Symposium on Multiple Personality. Edited by Braun BG. Psychiatr Clin North Am 7:121–134, 1984d

Kluft RP: The treatment of multiple personality disorder: current concepts, in Directions in Psychiatry (Volume 5). Edited by Flach FF. New York, Hatherleigh, 1985a

Kluft RP: Making the diagnosis of multiple personality disorder (MPD), in Directions in Psychiatry (Volume 5). Edited by Flach FF. New York, Hatherleigh, 1985b

Kluft RP: The natural history of multiple personality disorder, in Childhood Antecedents of Multiple Personality. Edited by Kluft RP. Washington, DC, American Psychiatric Press, 1985c

Kluft RP: Using hypnotic inquiry protocols to monitor treatment progress and stability in multiple personality disorder. Am J Clin Hypn 28:63–75, 1985d

Kluft RP, Braun BG, Sachs RG: Multiple personality, intrafamilial abuse, and family psychiatry. International Journal of Family Psychiatry 5:283–301, 1984

Kohlenberg RJ: Behavioristic approach to multiple personality: a case study. Behavior Therapy 4:137–140, 1973

Lampl-De Groot J: Notes on multiple personality. Psychoanal Q 50:614–624, 1981

Lasky R: The psychoanalytic treatment of a case of multiple personality. Psychoanal Rev 65:355–380, 1978

Levenson J, Berry S: Family intervention in a case of multiple personality. Journal of Marital and Family Therapy 9:73–80, 1983

Marmer SS: Psychoanalysis of multiple personality. Int J Psychoanal 61:439–459, 1980

Nemiah JC: Dissociative disorders, in Comprehensive Textbook of Psychiatry (Fourth Edition). Edited by Kaplan H, Sadock B. Baltimore, Williams and Wilkins, 1985

Orne MT, Dinges DF, Orne EC: On the differential diagnosis of multiple personality in the forensic context. Int J Clin Exp Hypn 32:118–169, 1984

Price J, Hess ND: Behavior therapy as a precipitant and treatment in a case of dual personality. Aust NZ J Psychiatry 13:63–66, 1979

Putnam FW: The study of multiple personality disorder: general strategies and practical considerations. Psychiatric Annals 14:58–61, 1984a

Putnam FW: The psychophysiological investigation of multiple personality disorder: a review, in Symposium on Multiple Personality. Edited by Braun BG. Psychiatr Clin North Am 7:31–39, 1984b

Putnam FW, Buchsbaum M, Howland F, et al: Evoked potentials in multiple personality disorder (New Research Abstract No. 139). Presented at the annual meeting of the American Psychiatric Association, Toronto, 1982

Putnam FW, Loewenstein RJ, Silberman EJ, et al: Multiple personality disorder in a hospital setting. J Clin Psychiatry 45:172–175, 1984

Putnam FW, Post RM, Guroff JJ, et al: One hundred cases of multiple personality disorder (New Research Abstract No. 77). Presented at the annual meeting of the American Psychiatric Association, New York, 1983

Schultz R, Braun BG, Kluft RP: Creativity and imaginary companion phenomena: prevalence and phenomenology in MPD, in Dissociative Disorders 1985: Proceedings of the Second International Conference on Multiple Personality/Dissociative States. Chicago, Rush University, 1985

Solomon RS, Solomon V: Differential diagnosis of multiple personality. Psychol Rep 51:1187–1194, 1982

Spanos NP, Weekes JR, Bertrand LD: Multiple personality: a social psychological perspective. J Abnorm Psychol 94:362–376, 1985

Spiegel D: Multiple personality disorder as a post-traumatic stress disorder, in Symposium on Multiple Personality. Edited by Braun BG. Psychiatr Clin North Am 7:101–110, 1984

Sutcliffe J, Jones J: Personal identity, multiple personality, and hypnosis. Int J Clin Exp Hypn 10:231–269, 1962

Taylor WS, Martin MF: Multiple personality. Journal of Abnormal and Social Psychology 39:281–300, 1944

Thigpen CH, Cleckley HM: On the incidence of multiple personality disorder: a brief communication. Int J Clin Exp Hypn 32:63–66, 1984

Victor G: Sybil: grand hysteria of folie a deux. Am J Psychiatry 132:202, 1974

Wilbur CG: Multiple personality and child abuse, in Symposium on Multiple Personality. Edited by Braun BG. Psychiatr Clin North Am 7:3–8, 1984

3

Dissociation, Double Binds, and Posttraumatic Stress in Multiple Personality Disorder

David Spiegel, M.D.

3

Dissociation, Double Binds, and Posttraumatic Stress in Multiple Personality Disorder

Two ubiquitous themes in the growing literature on multiple personality disorder (MPD) are a childhood history of severe, repeated physical trauma and the experience of uncontrolled dissociation (Bliss 1980; Braun 1985; Braun and Sachs 1985; Coons 1980; Kluft 1984, 1985; Prince 1905; Sutcliffe and Jones 1962; Spiegel 1984). Putnam (1986) found in a sample of 100 patients that 97 percent had been severely abused or neglected. Schultz et al. in 1985 found that 97.4 percent of 309 MPD patients in their study were also abused or neglected. From these findings, a theory of causation of MPD can be suggested. The model is that of unfortunate children who use dissociation as a defense, distancing themselves from the painful and frightening experience of abuse, but paying a heavy psychological price for this escape. These patients experience such extreme violation of their own internal physical and mental boundaries that they psychologically internalize this helplessness to control their physical world by coming to experience themselves as unable to control their own mental state, as they were unable to control their own lives or physically protect themselves. What early in life is a literal helplessness over their physical world becomes in later life a metaphorical helplessness over their psychological world. The unpredictability of parental assault becomes transformed into the unpredictability of the emergence of internalized parental objects. However, unlike borderline patients, who split external objects into good and bad, these dissociative disorder patients split internally. They are usually ruminative, depressed, and guilty about their early life experience, also unlike many borderline patients, who tend to be hostile, paranoid, and unable to tolerate dysphoria.

Trauma and Dissociation

The history of trauma in association with MPD is well documented. Wilbur (Wilbur 1984; Schreiber 1973) visited the home in which her famous patient, Sybil, was reared and found remnants of the equipment that had been used by Sybil's mother to torture the patient as a child. In addition, Kluft (1984) found a high prevalence of reports of physical and sexual abuse in the history of patients with MPD. He proposed a four-factor theory of etiology that includes 1) dissociation potential (as measured by hypnotizability); 2) life experience of severe trauma, which overwhelms the child's ego functioning; 3) ongoing dissociative phenomena such as imaginary companions, introjection, internalization, and identification, as well as social influences such as identification with a parent who has MPD; and 4) insufficient restorative experiences.

The interaction between childhood trauma and dissociation has received increasing attention. Fagan and McMahon (1984) described four cases in which children who were sexually abused demonstrated periods of dissociation and alternate personalities that resolved when the trauma was stopped and dealt with in psychotherapy. They noted the frequency of dissociative symptoms in children with MPD, including personality changes, forgetfulness, what appears to be a daze, and an overtly stoic attitude. Such dissociative symptoms are frequently unrecognized. For example, what would ordinarily be lying in a comparatively normal child is dissociation in a young MPD patient, who is then, of course, accused of lying or forgetting. Spiegel and Rosenfeld (1984) reported on an adolescent girl who dissociated not to an alternate personality with a different name but to herself at age four. When formally hypnotized, she could shift into this state and would begin crying, fearfully asking the examiner if he was going to hit her. She produced age-appropriate stick-figure drawings typical of a troubled four-year-old with no features on the faces and the figures of the child and the mother floating in the air (Spiegel and Spiegel 1985). It turned out that this girl had been beaten by her father just prior to her parents' divorce when she was 4 years old and subsequently had been raped by a baby sitter at age 8, raped by a photographer at age 12, and then forced into prostitution while working as a maid in a motel at age 15. When simple avoidance failed to separate her from this life, she began to dissociate openly and was hospitalized. There is thus accumulating evidence that dissociation is activated as a defense in childhood against sexual trauma or physical abuse and then continues to present itself as a symptom, especially if new trauma occurs.

The literature linking MPD to childhood history of trauma casts in a new light (Lipman 1985) an unexpected finding of Hilgard (1970) in her retrospective study of childhood experiences correlated with hypnotizability on the Stanford Hypnotic Susceptibility Scale: Form C. Hilgard was surprised by one variable that correlated .30 ($N = 187$) with hypnotizability. This variable was severity of punishment in childhood. The finding is especially important because it was counterintuitive to the investigator, who expected that support would enhance basic trust and hence hypnotizability. She found instead a persistent relationship between severe punishment and higher hypnotizability and speculated that "a possible tie between punishment and hypnotic involvement might come by way of dissociation. . . . Although we have no direct evidence, some of our case material . . . suggests that reading or other involvements may sometimes be an escape from the harsh realities of a punitive environment" (Hilgard 1970, p. 220). Thus, despite the absence of maternal warmth, children who had been severely punished tended to be more highly hypnotizable. Hilgard found this relationship between punishment and dissociation serendipitously in a homogeneous sample of socioeconomically privileged Stanford undergraduates, so the punishment–dissociation relationship could be expected to be even more vigorous among individuals who have suffered more extreme forms of discipline and outright abuse.

The organizing concept linking hypnotizability and trauma

in MPD is the victim's use of dissociation as a defense mechanism to control emotions in a dangerous situation and manage the subsequent pain and fear. One patient described it as "playing tricks with my mind" to control the pain. She would simply "leave," as she put it, by going to a mountain meadow full of wild flowers. She became expert at conducting routine conversations while dissociated, but eventually her sadistic father realized that she was emotionally absent from his sexual assaults and consciously attempted to hurt her so much that she could not "leave."

The repeated need to mobilize a dissociative defense tends to make its use habitual. Furthermore, it becomes incorporated into a cognitive framework. A patient preserves the integrity of his or her ego by dissociating it from the trauma, by saying "This did not happen to me." It happened to some dissociated and separate part of the self that in the extreme is identified as another personality. This position is reinforced by the amnesia that the person often consciously experiences for the details of the traumatic episode. These patients often experience a literal acting out of the worst fantasies that might be associated with a punitive and irrational superego. Frequently, parents rationalize the humiliation they inflict with statements that it is for the patient's own good, that he or she deserves it.

The parents' rationalization feeds into the other characteristic of dissociation, the patients' feeling of harboring the terrible secret that the real truth about themselves is that portion that was deservedly punished and damaged. Thus, the dissociation buys a certain temporary peace and perhaps survival at the time of abuse, at the price of an internal sense that the real self is the hidden one. They believe that whatever is true about them is unacceptable to the outside, adult world and it is all the worst aspects of the self. Because the repeated brutalization occurs during the period of preoperational thinking in the patients' cognitive development, the patients do not understand independent causation and therefore assume that they must have done something to elicit the response. However irrational it may be, this belief gives them a fantasy of control over events that render them helpless; that is, they can reassure themselves that if only they become a good girl or good boy, the beatings would stop.

THE DOUBLE BIND REVISITED

Despite repeated speculations about the etiological role of trauma in creating psychopathology, most such theories have foundered empirically, the best known example being Freud's (1905/1958) famous and recently debated recantation of the trauma theory as the etiology of neurosis. A more recent and no less vulnerable version of such theory is the double bind theory of the etiology of schizophrenia (Bateson 1972; Bateson et al. 1956). According to this theory, schizophrenic individuals' observed inability to correctly interpret meaning in the outside world, their resultant ambivalence, loose associations, and delusions, could be traced to deliberately confused messages (the double bind) inflicted on them by a parent. The double bind contains a primary injunction to the patient, along with a subtle secondary injunction that contradicts the first, and an unspoken but powerfully enforced rule that the paradox shall not be openly addressed. As an example, Bateson observed the peculiar response of a mother to her schizophrenic son's affectionate greeting:

> He was glad to see her and impulsively put his arm around her shoulders, whereupon she stiffened. He withdrew his arm and she asked, "Don't you love me anymore?" He then blushed, and she said, "Dear, you must not be so easily embarrassed and afraid of your feelings." (Bateson 1972, p. 217)

The double bind theory, although intriguing, collapsed under evidence for a biological/genetic component for schizophrenia (Kety et al. 1971) and development of the dopamine receptor hypersensitivity theory of the etiology of schizophrenia. The potency of neuroleptics in controlling the positive symptoms of schizophrenia such as delusions and hallucinations was found to be directly proportional to their ability to block dopamine receptors (Snyder 1976). Furthermore, the double bind and other theories of the etiology of schizophrenia, such as pseudomutuality (Wynne et al. 1958) and the concept of the schizophrenogenic parent (Lidz 1973), wound up being used more to scapegoat parents of schizophrenic children than to help treat or prevent the illness (Spiegel 1982). However, it may be that the theory died a premature death simply because it was applied to the wrong population of patients. Such extreme double bind communications are typical of parents of MPD patients. These physically abusive parents not infrequently rationalize their behavior to themselves and their children by telling them that they deserve the beating for some real or imagined transgression. The content of the message from the parent to the child is "I am good; you are bad," while the process of delivering it conveys the opposite about the parent. The child is of course terrorized into a reluctance to comment on the inherent paradox.

Although it is always dangerous to draw inferences about parental conduct on the basis of retrospective reports of patients, some personal experience with parents of MPD patients is consistent. For example, Mary, who had at least seven alternate personalities, was hospitalized because one personality, who had in earlier youth sheltered the patient from her father's sexual assaults, had determined that it was time for her to die. Indeed, the patient reported that her first memory of this alternate personality was when he summoned her to come and be with him the first time her father tied her to the bed with his neckties and raped her. When the patient reported the rape to her mother, the mother became enraged at her for daring to say such a thing about her father and permitted the sexual and physical abuse to continue for years. Indeed, the patient entered ongoing psychotherapy only after her father's death. The mother came to visit the patient during the hospitalization and was interviewed. Her manner was extremely formal and overtly polite and deferential (she repeatedly referred to the psychiatrist as "doctor") but the content of her comments conveyed exactly the opposite impression. She let it be known that she was a religious woman, that all problems could be handled through Scripture reading and religious practice, and that psychiatry was essentially a waste of time. When the psychiatrist commented on this apparent paradox, saying that "on the one hand you are extremely respectful and polite, and on the other hand you are conveying considerable disrespect for what I do," she nodded, smiled, and said, "Yes, that's right," utterly unruffled by the contradiction. In other cases, Drs. Bennett Braun and Richard Kluft have individually both received direct confirmation of paradox from the abuser (personal communication, Braun, March 1985).

Although in an acute sense the dissociation may be a defense against trauma, it may also represent a dramatic symbolic expression of the patient's response to the parent's demand that the patient be two contradictory people at the same time. That is what the patients indeed become. Frequently, the primary overt personality is rather dependent, passive, and painfully eager to please, and the first alternate personality is generally hostile, nonconformist, and noncompliant. This kind of dichotomy would well reflect the sort of double bind such patients experience from their parents. On one hand, they are always supposed to try to be good, absolutely perfect children, and on the other hand, both parents and children know the real truth, that the patients are bad, totally absorbed in their own desires, and utterly disrespectful of others. Thus, their response to the double bind imposed on them by their parents is to become the paradox, to become two or more discontinuous and conflicting people, and thus become all good, all bad, all cooperation, all defiance at the same time.

The third and all-important aspect of the double bind, that the victim is forbidden from commenting on the impossibility of his or her situation, is incorporated into the MPD patient as the impossibility of co-consciousness. Two conflicting personalities cannot coexist; their differences cannot be resolved. Sherry, for example, would compulsively respond to her mother's demand that she pay for the mother's household expenses by giving her her earnings, even though the mother was employed and had ample resources of her own. Routinely, the next day, an alternate personality would emerge when the patient was having lunch at a restaurant with her mother. She would walk to the bathroom, slit her wrist, and return to the table with blood dripping down her hand, giving her mother the vivid message, "You are bleeding me to death" and demonstrating that she was not the perfect compliant daughter the mother was asking her to be (Spiegel 1984).

Severe trauma inflicted by parents, as opposed to that inflicted by strangers, has elements of a macabre double bind. A beating or rape by a stranger, traumatic as it is, is in some ways easier to assimilate psychologically. It is a tragic event imposed from outside, seemingly for no reason. But rape by a father or physical abuse imposed by a mother has the bizarre quality of combining intense and longed-for attention from the parent with pain and humiliation. Furthermore, frequently the parents rationalize their behavior by telling children that it is "for your own good," will "whip you into shape," will "teach you what you need to know about life," and so on. Thus, these patients are left with intense and irreconcilable feelings, pain, fear, and humiliation on one hand and on the other the desire for something positive from their parents and the half-belief that the mistreatment is indeed for their own good. Furthermore, when such events happen in childhood, the victims have little ability to understand independent causation. They think in concrete terms and necessarily interpret what is done to them in light of their own conduct and role in eliciting it. They are made helpless to control both their own body and their own internal state. Indeed, highly hypnotizable patients have been observed to be especially vulnerable to outside cues while demonstrating a proneness to suspend their own critical scrutiny and internal sense of direction (Spiegel 1974). Such patients become structurally or spatially fragmented, unable to incorporate their history of trauma and conflicting parental messages into an acceptable unified sense of self. The defense against trauma becomes itself a source of distress.

TRAUMA AND FRAGMENTATION

When such trauma occurs at a later developmental state when independent causation can be understood, more frequently at the hands of a stranger, the standard dissociative defense is temporal fragmentation. Such a patient may forget a period of his or her life but may maintain a continuity of internal identity. For example, a 36-year-old Vietnam veteran with a 15-year service record suffered a fugue episode in which he wandered into the countryside in Vietnam, apparently ambushing Vietcong (Spiegel 1981). He finally returned to his base camp and was psychiatrically evacuated, placed on a series of antipsychotic and antidepressant medications, and variously diagnosed as schizophrenic and psychopathic, despite a previously unblemished military and psychiatric record. He became increasingly depressed and suicidal and was hospitalized in Army, Veterans Administration, and county psychiatric institutions for seven years. During the initial use of hypnotic regression with him, he relived for the first time the content of this amnesic episode:

He had discovered that an injured Vietnamese child whom he had adopted had been killed during the Tet Offensive. Seeing the boy's dead body triggered the fugue episode. The veteran relived with tremendous affect his finding and killing Vietcong and his tearful burial of his adopted son: "After 15 years in the Army, he was all I had. It's all my fault! It's all my fault! If I had just taken you over to the hooch, you wouldn't be there, man! It's not fair. They ain't gotta kill kids." This patient did not dissociate into alternative personalities, but the temporal fragmentation alone was sufficient to lead to a profound demoralization in which he came to believe that anything of value to him had died with his adopted son. The existence of the warded-off memories, relating both to his son's death and to his episode of vindictive revenge afterwards, was enough to undermine his sense of self and lead to a suicidal depression. This depression was resolved with psychotherapy aimed at helping him grieve the boy's loss while at the same time recalling and preserving the moments of joy that he had shared with his son. He was thus able to integrate into an acceptable view of himself the loss of the adopted son.

In MPD cases the trauma occurs earlier, is repeated, and is inflicted by loved ones. The sense of personal fragmentation is more profound, leading to the well-known fragmented self-concept. It is not merely the content of the alternative personalities that is of interest, but the personality structure, the sense of fragmentation, and the loss of control over consciousness that the uncontrolled dissociation entails. Any one self in an MPD patient is by definition incomplete, unacceptable, and out of control, never knowing when some other personality will emerge and take charge. Thus, the structure as well as the content of the disorder reflects the sense of helplessness and confused identity imposed on the patient.

PSYCHOTHERAPEUTIC CONSIDERATIONS

Multiple personality disorder can be conceptualized as a posttraumatic stress disorder that arises in response to repeated episodes of trauma imposed by hostile and double binding parents. Thus in planning the psychotherapy format, one can draw upon the literature on treatment of posttraumatic stress disorder and upon classical therapeutic principles (see Chapter 1).

Freud, in his paper, "Remembering, Repeating, and Working Through" (1914/1958), provided a major conceptual framework for psychotherapy. For MPD patients, memories of traumatic episodes may be accessible only in the context of certain dissociated states. The process of dissociation itself and the loss of control over consciousness is the repetition of the trauma, inviting working through in therapy. The patients repeat or reexperience their sense of physical helplessness through a psychological sense of helplessness to control consciousness.

As one might expect, the working through in therapy is complicated by transference considerations, in particular "traumatic transference." In this case, the patient unconsciously expects that the therapist, despite overt helpfulness and concern, will covertly exploit the patient for his or her own narcissistic gratification. Even therapeutic improvement is often attributed to the aggrandizement of the therapist rather than any genuine concern about the patient's improved well being. The patient of Spiegel and Rosenfeld (1984) who experienced spontaneous age regressions (described earlier in this chapter) reacted to the therapist as though he were her abusing father during the regression. She immediately cried and said "Please don't hit me." Because the regression was linked in her mind to an episode of abuse, she associated the therapist, because he was the person structuring her regression, with the abuse.

Accessing the memory, even for the purpose of working it through in therapy, is experienced as a reinflicting of previously experienced trauma, just as many rape victims experience police interrogation about the event as a repeat of the rape itself. Thus, the working through of transference is as difficult to resolve as it is critical. Furthermore, traditional analytic reserve is often perceived by the patient as a lack of concern or even sadistic pleasure in the patient's suffering. Such patients require active support and intervention, especially in dissociated episodes that have regressive components, such as when patients are reliving an assault as a child. They need the kind of structured supportive interaction that a child would need.

Treatment of MPD must involve a reintegration of the traumatized aspects of the self into an acceptable overall self-image. This can be done in traditional uncovering psychotherapy as long as the therapy focuses on the recollection of traumatic events and their meaning for the patient. Hypnosis can be a useful tool in facilitating this process. Because these patients dissociate anyway, hypnosis provides a convenient means of demonstrating their ability to induce dissociations into alternative personality states or to age regress to specific traumatic episodes, while teaching them control over the transitions. This is especially important because the loss of control is a key issue in trauma and, therefore, in these patients' lives. They expect to be made helpless when asked to undergo hypnosis. For some patients, fragmenting into a series of personalities is an attempt at separation and individuation. They maintain a sense of separateness by having secret personalities who are experienced as independent of parental control. Indeed, these patients often enhance their sense of control by identifying with the aggressor, the abusive parent. One or more of the dissociated personalities often inflicts physical harm in the same way that the parent did, conveying a false sense of mastery over the physical abuse.

These intense episodes can be used productively to help the patients experience their fear and helplessness and identify those feelings as a source of their disorganization and at the same time interweave dysphoric memories and affects into an acceptable and more integrated view of self by reliving their courage in trying to preserve themselves. When it was pointed out to Spiegel and Rosenfeld's (1984) age-regressing patient that she had shown considerable courage in trying to protect her mother from her father, she was surprised to think of herself as brave rather than simply terrified. She simultaneously came to experience her subsequent practice of self-hypnosis as a "protective light" surrounding her. She was able to balance her sense of helplessness with a recognition of her own courage in facing the endless fear that was her childhood.

Another organizing concept that is quite helpful in the psychotherapy of MPD patients is grief work. The process of working through the traumatic experience involves grieving a variety of losses: of self-image, of an idealized image of the abusing parent, of siblings hurt or killed. This conceptualization is based on Lindemann's (1944) description of grief work necessary for coming to terms with traumatic losses. Multiple personality patients often protect an image of their parents at their own expense. This unwillingness to relinquish a sense of personal responsibility for events inflicted on them by sadistic parents is at one level a sensible desire to avoid antagonizing an already cruel parent projecting a sense of badness onto the child. At another level, similar to the response of adults who are subjected to sudden trauma, it is an unconscious effort to experience control rather than helplessness in the face of adversity. The fantasy of potential undoing of trauma is a powerful incentive, despite the cost in self-esteem. Later on, such patients act helpless and relinquish opportunities to control their lives to keep alive the fantasy that they could have prevented or controlled their previous victimization. The therapeutic work involves grieving artificial images of parental perfection.

Intervention strategies for handling trauma within the therapy of MPD can be summarized with eight principles:

Confront trauma. It is important to identify traumatic origins of dissociation and personality fragmentation. Failure to identify these issues will reinforce patients' belief in their being bad and deserving the misery inflicted on them. Although obviously some of these memories may be fantasy rather than reality—indeed highly hypnotizable individuals are frequently unable to distinguish vivid fantasies from reality—it is important in therapy to take recollections of trauma seriously and use them as organizing concepts for working through childhood antecedents of current symptomatology.

Find a condensation of the traumatic experience. Often traumatic episodes are emotionally overwhelming to patient and therapist alike; it is helpful to find some image that condenses the experience and makes it available to memory but manageable.

There must often be a period of confession. The patient may need to confess to some moment of terror, sense of cowardice, or overwhelming desire for revenge against a parent.

Consolation is important. The therapist must demonstrate empathic concern for the patient and provide a balanced view, integrating the overwhelming affect of the patient into a conceptual framework that does not minimize any real lapses on the part of the patient but puts them into a broader context, balancing the patient's strong points and weak points.

Make conscious previously repressed or dissociated material. Gradually, material that is initially recalled only in a dossociated state must be worked into one increasingly unified consciousness.

Guide concentration to the development of an integrated view of self. The integrated view of the self must incorporate conflicting images elicited by traumatic as well as normal experiences. Hypnosis is often useful in helping the patient focus on such images.

Control. Hypnotic age regression may help to unearth previous memories and control emotional reactions. This therapeutic work must be conducted in such a way that it gives the patient an enhanced sense of control over unbidden images and hence over alternative personality states.

Congruence. The ultimate goal is to help the patient face and bear a period of tragedy and integrate it into their ongoing life.

These principles have proved useful in the psychotherapy of patients who have posttraumatic stress disorder and those who have MPD. The latter indeed are doubly bound, by parental communication that included trauma and by dissociation that started as a defense but became a symptom. Frequently MPD patients symbolize as internal fragmentation the cruel paradox of sadistic mistreatment in the guise of parental concern. The familiar double bind becomes the internal multiplicity of personalities. The need to endure pain and fear becomes uncontrolled dissociation. Effective treatment requires recognition of these traumatic origins and active collaboration with the patients to identify and control dissociation in the service of unbinding them from their traumatic past.

REFERENCES

Bateson G: Steps to an Ecology of Mind. New York, Ballantine Books, 1972

Bateson G, Jackson D, Haley J, et al: Toward a theory of schizophrenia. Behav Sci 1:251–264, 1956

Bliss EL: Multiple personalities: a report of 14 cases with implications for schizophrenia and hysteria. Arch Gen Psychiatry 37:1388–1397, 1980

Braun BG: The transgenerational incidence of dissociation and multiple personality disorder: a preliminary report, in Childhood Antecedents of Multiple Personality. Edited by Kluft RP. Washington, DC, American Psychiatric Press, 1985

Braun BG, Sachs RG: The development of multiple personality disorder: predisposing, precipitating and perpetuating factors, in Childhood Antecedents of Multiple Personality. Edited by Kluft RP. Washington, DC, American Psychiatric Press, 1985

Coons PM: Multiple personality: diagnostic considerations. Journal of Clinical Psychiatry 41:330–336, 1980

Fagan J, McMahon PP: Incipient multiple personality in children. J Nerv Ment Dis 172:26–35, 1984

Freud S: A case of hysteria, three essays on sexuality, and other works. Volume 7, The Standard Edition of the Complete Psychological Works of Sigmund Freud. London, Hogarth, 1958

Freud S: Remembering, repeating, and working-through (further recommendations on the technique of psycho-analysis II). Volume 12, The Standard Edition of the Complete Psychological Works of Sigmund Freud. London, Hogarth, 1958

Hilgard JR: Personality and Hypnosis: A Study of Imaginative Involvement. Chicago, University of Chicago Press, 1970

Kety SS, Rosenthal, D, Wender PH, et al: Mental illness in the biological and adoptive families of adopted schizophrenics. Am J Psychiatry 128:82–86, 1971

Kluft RP: Treatment of multiple personality disorder, in Symposium on Multiple Personality. Edited by Braun BG. Psychiatr Clin North Am 7:9–29, 1984

Kluft RP: Childhood multiple personality disorder: predictors, clinical findings and treatment results, in Childhood Antecedents of Multiple Personality. Edited by Kluft RP. Washington, DC, American Psychiatric Press, 1985

Lidz T: The Origin and Treatment of Schizophrenic Disorders. New York, Basic Books, 1973

Lindemann E: Symptomatology and management of acute grief. Am J Psychiatry 101:141–148, 1944

Lipman LS: Hypnotizability and multiple personality. Presented at the annual meeting of the American Psychiatric Association, Dallas, 1985

Prince M: The Dissociation of a Personality. London, Longmans, Green, 1905

Putnam FW, Guroff JJ, Silberman EK, et al: The clinical phenomenology of multiple personality disorder: 100 recent cases. Journal of Clinical Psychiatry 47:285–293, 1986

Schreiber FR: Sybil. Chicago, Henry Regnery, 1973

Schultz R, Braun BG, Kluft RP: Creativity and imaginary companion phenomena: prevalence and phenomenology in MPD, in Dissociative Disorders 1985: Proceedings of the Second International Conference on Multiple Personality/Dissociative States. Edited by Braun BG. Chicago, Rush University, 1985

Snyder SH: The dopamine hypothesis of schizophrenia: focus on the dopamine receptor. Am J Psychiatry 133:197–202, 1976

Spiegel D: Vietnam grief work using hypnosis. Am J Clin Hypn 24:33–40, 1981

Spiegel D: Mothering, fathering, and mental illness, in Rethinking the Family: Some Feminist Questions. Edited by Thorne B, Yalom M. New York, Longman, 1982

Spiegel D: Multiple personality as a post-traumatic stress disorder, in Symposium on Multiple Personality. Edited by Braun BG. Psychiatr Clin North Am 7:101–110, 1984

Spiegel D, Rosenfeld A: Spontaneous hypnotic age regression. Journal of Clinical Psychiatry 45:522–524, 1984

Spiegel D, Spiegel H: Hypnosis, in Comprehensive Textbook of Psychiatry (Volume 4). Edited by Kaplan HI, Sudeck BJ. Williams and Wilkins, 1985

Spiegel H: The Grade 5 syndrome: the highly hypnotizable person. Inter J Clin Exp Hypn 22:303–319, 1974

Sutcliffe JP, Jones J: Personal identity, multiple personality, and hypnosis. Int J Clin Exp Hypn 10:231–269, 1962

Wilbur CB: Multiple personality and child abuse, in Symposium on Multiple Personality. Edited by Braun BG. Psychiatr Clin North Am 7:3–8, 1984

Wynne L, Ryckoff E, Day J, et al: Pseudomutuality in the family relations of schizophrenics. Psychiatry 21:205–220, 1958

4

Treating Children Who Have Multiple Personality Disorder

Richard P. Kluft, M.D.

4

Treating Children Who Have
Multiple Personality Disorder

Multiple personality disorder (MPD) has long been considered a psychopathology of childhood origin and onset. Until recently, however, there was little documentation to sustain this assumption. What evidences were available were drawn from lay accounts and the reports of patients in therapy. Inevitably, these reports were anecdotal and retrospective. It remained uncertain whether MPD existed among younger patients in either a classical or a nascent form, whether some developmental process of uncertain duration gradually transformed some precursors of MPD into the adult condition (which is usually first diagnosed between the ages of 20 and 40 years), or even whether MPD had no antecedents other than therapists' and patients' inadvertent or willful encouragement of the enactment of MPD behaviors (Kluft 1984a, 1985a).

For almost 140 years, the only report of MPD in a child was Despine's study of "Estelle," a girl of 11, which was published in 1840. Despite Ellenberger's extensive summary of the Despine study in his encyclopedic *The Discovery of the Unconscious* (1970), Despine's work remained relatively unknown in the MPD field. The original study is absent from Boor and Coons's (1983) and Damgaard, Van Benschoten, and Fagan's (1985) bibliographies of the literature relevant to MPD. However, Despine has influenced my clinical work (1984a, 1985a, 1985b) with childhood MPD, and I credit him with inspiring my case-finding research.

I have been unable to find any retrievable references to childhood MPD cases between 1840 and 1979; nor could Fagan and McMahon (1984) or Dr. Philip M. Coons, who kindly reviewed his own voluminous materials (personal communication, June 1983), find any. Since 1979, however, the study of childhood cases of MPD has become one of many new areas of exploration among recent efforts to advance psychiatric understanding of the dissociative disorders. In 1979, I reported the diagnosis and successful treatment of MPD in an eight-year-old boy in a course at the annual meeting of the American Psychiatric Association. This case was noted in passing in a 1982 treatment article (Kluft 1982). In the same year, Elliott (1982) argued that the diagnosis of MPD in a child should prompt state intervention on the grounds of probable child abuse. She reported that several clinicians she had polled in the course of her research had encountered cases of MPD in children. Also in 1982, Weiss, Sutton, and Utecht presented their work with a 10-year-old girl who was suffering from MPD to the American Academy of Child Psychiatry. Two years later (1984a) I reported five cases of DSM-III-classified (*Diagnostic and Statistical Manual of Mental Disorders* [*Third Edition*]; American Psychiatric Association 1980) MPD in children and then elaborated on my findings in further accounts (1985a, 1985b). Two of these cases were transgenerational: one patient was the son of an MPD parent; another was the son of two MPD parents. The latter case was trigenerational—the mother's mother also had MPD. Fagan and McMahon (1984) described less structured dissociative conditions of childhood as "incipient multiple personality," drawing attention to the probability that precursors to well-defined MPD could be identified and treated. Weiss et al.'s work was published in 1985. Confirmation of my finding of a generational quality to some cases of MPD was provided by Braun's (1985) extensive study of 18 families and Coons's (1985) anterospective study, in which an MPD youngster was found among the children of MPD parents. These studies document the existence of MPD patients who are at greater than average risk for developing MPD.

At the time of this writing, approximately 20 colleagues have informed me of more than 50 childhood cases of MPD. Those do not include cases of "incipient MPD." The importance of the identification of these cases for the study of MPD is difficult to overstate. Although a detailed exploration of the implications of these findings falls outside the scope of this chapter, a few observations and comments may be presented.

Findings regarding MPD in children are largely consistent with the retrospective accounts of adult MPD patients. This suggests that MPD patients' accounts of past mistreatment, no matter how repugnant or straining to the clinician's credulity, should be taken quite seriously and explored with an awareness that therapists often experience profound pressures to disavow and discredit accounts that actually may be mainly accurate or that may prove to be screen memories hiding real traumata (Goodwin 1985). Most of the childhood cases thus far reported support the etiological importance accorded to child abuse, long considered a common if not universal antecedent to MPD (Wilbur 1984). Putnam et al. (1985) found that 97 percent of 100 MPD patients (reported by 92 therapists) had experienced mistreatment during childhood. Schultz et al. (1985) found that 97 percent of 307 MPD patients (reported by 309 therapists) had experienced forms of child abuse. In one published instance (1984a, 1985a, 1985b) and a second unpublished instance, I serendipitously assessed youngsters who had not experienced abuse and found no evidence of MPD. Reassessment of these children after documented and confessed abuse revealed them to have classic MPD. However, it is now clear that abuse is not invariably present. Cases with dissociation due to other etiologies have been described, including object loss, object loss and loss of numerous caretakers, near-death experience, exposure to death, accidental gunshot wound, and autohypnotic withdrawal from family chaos (Kluft 1984b and unpublished data).

Childhood cases also facilitate confirmation or disconfirmation of theories that have been put forth on the basis of the study of adult cases. Many authors have suggested that MPD is a borderline variant and that the personalities develop on a substrate of failures of cohesion of self and object representations. Many childhood cases do not seem to have problems in that area (Kluft 1984a), suggesting that dissociative "splitting" and splitting as it is described in the psychoanalytic literature are not identical processes. The findings in children are more consistent with the research of Horevitz and Braun (1984), who discovered that although many MPD patients also qualified for a borderline diagnosis, many did not. This suggests that the two conditions are different but may coexist. Taken as a whole, the limited findings currently available from childhood MPD cases suggest that MPD is the final common pathway for many possible combinations of etiological factors and that theories that do not account for this have limited generalizability, even if they do accurately capture the dynamics of a given individual case. Formulations offered by Kluft (1984b) and by Braun and Sachs (1985) have sufficient breadth to accommodate the numerous etiological combinations that may place a given patient on the MPD pathway.

The cases studied thus far offer an encouraging prognosis for the treatment of MPD in children. The childhood patients reported in the literature have recovered, usually with celerity, and retained their gains. I have followed two successfully integrated patients for seven and four years respectively. Instruments, although crude and unvalidated, already are available for screening children for MPD (Fagan and McMahon 1984; Kluft 1984a; Putnam [in Kluft 1984a]). These instruments are not diagnostic, but they suggest which children should be carefully assessed for MPD by an experienced clinician. A more rigorous and refined protocol is under development by Putnam (personal communication, October 1985). Whereas adult MPD is associated with considerable suffering and usually requires extensive treatment (Kluft 1984b), incipient and childhood MPD is usually treated rapidly, and the child is enabled to resume normal growth and development (Kluft 1984a). It is desirable and it should be possible to mount energetic efforts to identify and treat MPD in its childhood forms and thus prevent the development of the more entrenched adult condition. This would reduce the suffering and incapacity of those afflicted with MPD and spare their loved ones and society the burdens of their morbidity and the costs attendant upon their care. It might also interdict the transgenerational passage of MPD.

In this chapter, the available literature on the treatment of children who have MPD is reviewed and augmented with thoughtful observations from approximately 20 colleagues involved with such cases. From this body of experience, a preliminary treatment overview and an outline of what appears to be useful in work with such patients are presented. It is acknowledged that this synthesis is undertaken at a point in time when all findings are preliminary and tentative and thus is likely to require substantial revision after future investigations. An overall description of childhood MPD and the general principles of the treatment of adults with MPD are beyond the scope of this chapter. For a description of childhood MPD, the reader is referred to reports by Kluft (1984a, 1985a, 1985b, 1985c), Fagan and McMahon (1984), and Weiss et al. (1985). For a discussion of general issues in the treatment of MPD, the reader is referred to the following special issues of journals that were dedicated to MPD: Issue 2 of Volume 26 of the *American Journal of Clinical Hypnosis* (October 1983), Issue 1 of Volume 14 of *Psychiatric Annals* (January 1984), and Issue 1 of Volume 7 of *Psychiatric Clinics of North America* (March 1984). A recent comprehensive review (Kluft 1985c) is also available that excerpts the classic treatment advices of Bowers et al. (1971) and Braun's description of the stages of therapy for MPD (1980; also see Chapter 1 in this monograph).

LITERATURE REVIEW

A literature search revealed 10 references to the treatment of MPD in childhood. In two, the treatment of childhood cases is merely noted without further elaboration (Kluft 1982, 1984b).

Despine's original work (1840) is difficult to retrieve. The contemporary reader usually must rely on Ellenberger's account (1970). Despine undertook to treat an 11-year-old Swiss girl, Estelle, believed to be paralyzed by a spinal cord lesion. She suffered excruciating pains, hallucinations, and visions and often seemed oblivious to her surroundings. After months of slow improvement under a regimen of hydrotherapy and electrotherapy, Estelle's mother told Despine that Estelle was comforted by angels. He began to suspect a "magnetic," that is, hypnotic, pathology. After some negotiation over control issues and Estelle's reluctance to accept hypnosis, she proved to be a good subject. A protector and helper personality—a comforting angel—was found. This entity, Angeline, imposed certain conditions on the treatment but was generally constructive and cooperative. Within a month, Estelle remained her proper but distressed self in the waking state, but in another state, elicited by hypnosis, she was able to walk and was far less deferential. Soon the states were emerging spontaneously. After several months the patient predicted she would visualize a huge ball, that it would burst, and that improvement would follow. This came to pass and heralded Estelle's being able to walk in the state in which previously she had been paralyzed. Within two months, her symptoms were resolved and her separate states fused. Ellenberger composed a concise formulation of the therapeutic principles that informed the efforts of the "magnetizers" of Despine's era (1970).

I have contended (1984a) that Despine implicitly anticipated many of the approaches and ideas now finding wide acceptance in the treatment of MPD. Despine was open to reconsider the diagnosis when the patient's response to standard therapy was suboptimal. He included magnetic, that is, hypnotic, pathologies within differential diagnosis. Therefore, neither her quasipsychotic symptoms nor her pseudoorganicity consigned Estelle to misdiagnosis. He approached her gradually and carefully, mobilizing her strengths and assets to assist the therapeutic process. He remained respectful and nonjudgmental, even when his authority was challenged. He recognized that Estelle's family played a part in her situation. When Despine encountered separate entities or states, he neither denied or suppressed them nor minimized their importance. He allowed them to express themselves, noted their differences, and avoided intrusiveness and skepticism. He managed his patient's misgivings about hypnosis by negotiating terms under which she could accept such interventions, an early example of contracting. Clearly, Despine understood the concept of therapeutic alliance. He paced the treatment with what he learned from Estelle, from the more outspoken "hypnotic Estelle," and from Angeline. He learned to avoid unnecessary power struggles, narcissistic clashes, and confrontations with Angeline. Even when she was grandiose, Despine worked toward collaboration. His use of hypnosis was judicious. He accepted and worked with Estelle's autohypnotic imagery, especially her metaphor for fusion. He tolerated the different behavioral styles of the separate states in a manner that facilitated Estelle's dealing with her problems with enmeshment, dependency, and authority.

I undertook an exegesis of Despine's approach before I encountered childhood cases of MPD. My methods in treating childhood MPD (Kluft 1984a, 1985a, 1985b; Kluft et al. 1984) are influenced by Despine and informed by my four-factor theory of the etiology of MPD, derived from study of adult cases (1984b). After several years of attempting to comprehend and explain MPD on the basis of object relations and self-psychology models, I concluded that although such formulations might accurately reflect the mental structures of occasional MPD patients, they could not be generalized to all cases. I was particularly impressed that some MPD patients' alternate personalities fused rapidly and permanently after abreaction alone and that their previously separate identifying characteristics blended with those of the personalities with whom they fused, yielding a configuration encompassing findings in both fusion partners. Some patients completely integrated very rapidly on this basis and were sustaining their fusion upon follow-up. I also found that many phenomena suggestive of borderline pathology in MPD resolved far more rapidly than similar phenomena in conventional borderline patients. Because this observation was inconsistent with the arduous efforts necessary to change preoedipal pathologies in psychoanalytic psychotherapy treatments, I reasoned that despite superficial similarities, the "splitting" attributed to MPD patients was a different phenomenon from the splitting observed in borderline pathologies. It thus seemed unrealistic to assume that basic failures of integration of self and object representation could be corrected on the basis of a few sessions' work or would respond to hypnotic fusion rituals. The four-factor theory, therefore, regards preoedipal failures of integration of self and object representations as one among many potential contributions to MPD organization, but it does not conceptualize such pathology as inherent to the MPD condition. Horevitz and Braun's recent (1984) study offers empirical substantiation for this formulation.

The four-factor theory postulates that every patient who develops MPD has four factors in his or her constitution, experience, intrapsychic organization, and interpersonal environment. It was formed from a retroactive review of 73 cases in 1979 and has been studied anterospectively on more than 150 cases since then. Thus far it appears robust and flexible and inclusive enough to encompass virtually all plausible speculations as to the origin of MPD.

Factor 1 of the four-factor theory is the biological capacity to dissociate, or dissociation potential. This was initially understood as the biologic but not the compliance or suggestibility component of hypnotizability (Spiegel and Spiegel 1978). It has been validated by documentation from Bliss (1983, 1984a, 1984b), Lipman et al. (1984), and Lipman (1985) that MPD patients are a highly hypnotizable group of patients. De Vito (1984) suggested postulating a fifth factor to encompass other psychobiological substrates that may be found (personal communication, 1985) or enlarging the understanding of Factor 1, dissociation potential, to include other biologic mechanisms of dissociation, possibly based on ictal events or neurotransmitter alterations.

Factor 2 encompasses life experiences that traumatically overwhelm the nondissociative defensive/adaptive aspects of the child's ego. Clearly, the most common vehicle of such experiences is child abuse (Putnam et al. 1985; Schultz et al. 1985). I have listed nonabuse etiologies (1984b, 1985a), and the young lady discussed by Weiss et al. (1985) appears to have dissociated in response to object loss and numerous changes of her primary caretakers. The theory specifies that certain factors may weaken the patient's resilience, and thus events or circumstances that would appear to be of lesser traumatic potential are able to precipitate dissociation into separate personalities. Problems in the process of separation and individuation, difficulties in achievement of cohesive self and object representations, and the impact of congenital anomalies may lower a child's resistance to dissociative dividedness under stress. Indeed, Weiss et al.'s (1985) patient had many abnormalities, probably attributable to fetal alcohol syndrome.

Factor 3 is the presence of shaping influences and substrates that determine the form taken by the dissociative defenses. Unable to find a developmental or psychodynamic commonality across my patients, I postulated that in each case a unique configuration of intrapsychic structures and dynamics and environmental influences had converged to give rise to the phenomenological expression of MPD. Hence it is difficult to generalize about the structure, the treatment, and the prognosis of the disorder.

Factor 4 is the inadequate provision of stimulus barriers and restorative experiences. I hypothesized that the conjunction of Factors 1–3 was relatively frequent but that MPD, although more common than generally recognized, was still less frequently encountered than would be predicted if Factors 1–3 invariably produced MPD. Dissociation is a reasonably common defense in overwhelmed children, and many separatenesses, initiated by trauma, are healed by soothing, restorative experiences. If a traumatized child who dissociated and developed a separateness were protected, nurtured, and helped to process his or her hurt, the necessity for the dividedness would be eroded, and unity might well be restored. Conversely, if such a child were further abused, and/or received minimal consolation or soothing, and/or was not encouraged to deal with his or her painful experiences, and/or was given double-binding communications about what had happened, the need for the dissociative defense would remain, and the development of MPD as a stable adaptation would be encouraged. I predicted that when MPD children were discovered, interventions based on Factor 4—treatment focused on removing the need for the ongoing use of dissociative defenses—would have a high likelihood of success. Braun and Sachs (1985) reached similar conclusions in their discussion of the predisposing, precipitating, perpetuating factors of MPD, as did Albini and Schwartz (1985), who speculated that Factor 4 failures might force the patient to mobilize Factor 3 substrates for self-soothing, a formulation analogous in many respects to a psychoanalytic developmental theory explicated by Marmer (1980).

I have successfully treated four children with MPD (see Kluft 1984, 1985a, 1985b; Kluft et al. 1984). In the case of Tommy, whose parents and maternal grandmother proved to have MPD, I intervened with the parents and insisted they intervene at school in order to interdict abuse, relieve pressure on the child, and make it possible for the child's academic potential to be reassessed. Using techniques successful with adults (Kluft 1982), I gained access to the boy's alter personalities with hypnosis, helped them verbalize their concerns and abreact their experiences, listened to them empathically, and worked toward their reconciliation. Finally, I used hypnotically facilitated imagery techniques to age-progress the personalities to a common age and then to encourage integration. After integration, working through, finding alternative approaches to dysfunctional coping styles, and stabilizing gains were promoted. I have followed up on the patient at regular intervals for the last seven years.

Another case involved a dysfunctional boy, Bobby, who was determined to deny his abuse experience and had a personality who tried to evade discovery. I involved child welfare workers and the legal system to supervise, help, and control an abusive parent. Through hypnosis I was able to gain access to the alter personality (Kluft 1982) and enlisted the contrite abuser to give the boy permission to be honest about the abuse and to support him in facing his traumatic experiences. Fusion was followed by rerepression of the traumata; these were recovered through hypnotic techniques such as age regression. I insisted on certain contingencies to support the boy's recovery: the abuser's cooperation with me and with the child welfare workers, therapy for the abuser, and an understanding that a resumption of abuse would lead to immediate hospitalization. The abuse was repeated, and the abuser was hospitalized. Seen within a week of the repeated abuse, the boy had developed a new personality, an identification with the abuser. Treatment was successful. As a guard against recidivism, I insisted on ongoing supervision by child welfare personnel until all children in the family graduate from high school. This youngster has now sustained integration for more than four years.

In another case, a multidisciplinary team used family therapy, individual treatment of the child and the family members, the structure of a hospital milieu, and hypnotic intervention by a consultant to treat a suicidal MPD youngster named Otto. Another youngster integrated after the alleviation of environmental pressures via family interventions. Details of the family interventions used in these cases are described by Kluft et al. (1984).

Fagan and McMahon (1984) treated their patients Sara and Cindy with family therapy and individual therapy for both children and the adopting (nonabusive) parents. When findings suggested previous abuse, a caseworker documented that this had occurred. Play therapy was structured to allow the girls to reenact their abuse experience with dolls. This precipitated abreactive events in and outside of the sessions, followed by a cessation of dissociative symptoms. Their patient Susan was treated with play therapy. Dolls and role play were used to

explore the patient's two personalities and effect their reconciliation, and an imagery technique was used to bring about
fusion. It was used without hypnosis. Tom, a four-year-old, was
treated in play therapy and responded rapidly. Their patient
Ellen was an adolescent, 14 years of age. They did not specify
their therapeutic approach in this case, which proved unsuccessful.

Fagan and McMahon (1984) outlined treatment plans for
children with MPD on the basis of the family's level of function
and cooperativeness and the child's age and severity of allo-
plastic behaviors. They defined supportive families as those
with nonabusing parents who have minimal personal pathology
and a commitment to treatment. Treatment for an MPD child
from a supportive family would be play therapy augmented by
family therapy to support the parents and their relationship
and help them deal with the child. Problematic families were
defined as those no longer abusing the child but having pathological features that stress the child and evoke (and thereby
strengthen) the protecting and defending personalities. The
parents may be too preoccupied to attend to the child or may
overtly reject the child. The treatment they prescribed for an
MPD child in such a family is, if the parents will cooperate, a
combination of individual, couple, and family therapy, plus
treatment for the child. If the parents are uncooperative, the
intercession of child welfare workers is necessary, along with
assessment as to whether the children should be placed in care
outside the home. They suggest that the first priority is the
detoxification of the family environment. Until this is achieved,
the child must be treated supportively. To open up the child
prior to establishing his or her safety could be dangerous. With
pathological families, severe abuse of the MPD child is ongoing,
and one or both parents are quite ill. One may be unaware that
the other is an abuser and/or serves as an enabler of the abuse.
If the abuser is mentally ill, he or she should be treated, possibly
in the hospital. Some abusers might profit from specialized
groups for abusers. The nonabusive parents may require support groups. Fagan and McMahon were unable to offer generalizations about this group.

Fagan and McMahon emphasize that whereas children often
can be managed as outpatients, adolescents may have acting
out and suicidal behaviors that require the structure of an in-

patient setting. They recommend a modification of Greaves's (1980) approaches to adult patients. They advocate a therapeutic stance of gentle power, honesty, and acceptance, with listening as the most important therapeutic activity. Exploration is via fantasy, therapeutic games, drawing, sculpting, and story telling. They advise making the personalities quite tangible, helping them meet their needs constructively, and beginning to move toward alliance, working on issues of trust and mistrust. They recommend that the therapist present past traumata in symbolic forms via play materials, encouraging abreaction and the taking of assertive and masterful actions in the fantasies, dealing actively with situations in which the child had once been a passive victim. During this process more memories emerge, and feelings spill over outside therapy hours. Parents, teachers, and others must be helped to anticipate and manage this phase. After abreaction, integration is pursued by fantasy age progression and fusion fantasies. Postintegration treatment solidifies gains, identifies new strengths, and works on residual and newly emergent problems. The major differences between Fagan and McMahon's (1984) approach and mine (1984a, 1985a, 1985b) are as follows: 1) I occasionally used formal hypnosis, whereas Fagan and McMahon preferred imagery techniques without formal hypnosis; 2) Fagan and McMahon tried to concretize the personalities, and I meticulously avoided doing so; and 3) Fagan and McMahon used play therapy techniques, which I did not use. It is difficult to determine the substance of these differences. My child patients averaged 8.5 years of age; Fagan and McMahon's four children averaged 5.5 years of age. My patients responded well to standard verbal therapy. Had my patients been younger, I might well have used play therapy techniques. In view of the trance proneness of such patients, it is possible that imagery techniques evoked trance phenomena. It is also possible that although Fagan and McMahon's (1984) wording suggests the concretization of personalities as a therapeutic technique per se, in fact the article suggests it may have been used to provide the structure of the characterizations of the doll participants in the play therapy.

Weiss et al. (1985) treated their patient in a hospital setting. The milieu controlled unacceptable behaviors and encouraged appropriate ones. Calming medications were used. The girl's adoptive parents were involved in supportive casework treatment. Twenty months of verbal psychotherapy alone failed to control self-abuse, relieve amnesia, or bring about integration. Consequently, hypnosis was used. It permitted exploration of incidents and clarification of motivations, encouragement of adaptive behaviors and self-control, and a constructive dialogue among the personalities. Amnestic barriers were eroded; repressed memories were recovered, abreacted, and worked through. Her troublesome behaviors changed toward more appropriate patterns, and the phenomena of MPD faded away.

SYNOPSIS OF REPORTED TREATMENT STRATEGIES

The therapists who report successful treatment of childhood MPD have been able to control their patients' life space so as to protect the children from further traumatization by others and from self-inflicted harm. This has involved 1) reporting abuse and cooperating collaboratively with child protective workers, 2) setting firm limits with abusers and enforcing them scrupulously, and 3) refusing to enter collusions that might replicate the face-saving falsehoods of the abusing family's pseudonormal veneer (Kluft et al. 1984) or perpetuate the ersatz realities that Summit (1983) described as the "child abuse accommodation syndrome." They have used hospitalization to control aggressive and self-destructive behaviors.

These therapists have protected the children as well by declining to begin exploratory work until the overall treatment is secured. I recommend videotaping initial assessments when it appears likely that abusers will deny their abuse and/or that hypnotic or other treatments might be held to have contaminated the child's credibility later as a witness. Guidelines used for forensic hypnosis (Orne 1979) are recommended.

Successful therapists have discovered that it is crucial to deal with the child's painful experiences—treatment based on improving social skills alone is at best a partial remedy. They have discovered means of gaining access to these experiences when the child cannot and/or will not discuss them. Because undirected interventions may fail to reach the painful areas that must be explored, these therapists do not hesitate to intervene rather actively. Weiss et al. (1985) achieved more in five months with the use of hypnosis than they had in the prior 20 months of conversational therapy. Fagan and McMahon (1984) used data from ancillary sources to create play scenarios that brought about their patients' abreactions of traumata. I used hypnotic techniques early in the treatment of most cases (1984a, 1985a, 1985b).

It is clear that with controlled, protected, and active treatments child MPD patients usually recover unity rather rapidly and that the length of time required to achieve unity may be age-related. Fagan and McMahon's (1984) patients, averaging 5.5 years of age, improved within a few sessions. My patients, averaging 8.5 years of age, recovered unity within 15 or fewer sessions (1984a, 1985a, 1985b). For Weiss et al. (1985), who did not begin hypnotherapy until their patient, Laura, was approximately 12 years of age, 30 sessions were required over a period of five months to help her unify.

Of course, achieving unification is only one aspect of patients' treatments. Successful therapies also include treatment of families that are appropriate to retain their MPD children. This includes family therapy, work with subsystems of the family, individual treatment of its members on occasion, and referral for specialized group experiences for some. It stands to reason than an MPD child, if returned to an environment unchanged from the one that precipitated and/or perpetuated the development of MPD, is condemned to relapse or worse.

ANECDOTAL EXPERIENCES

Since my first description of a case of childhood MPD in 1979, I have had more than 200 contacts with clinicians or other concerned individuals who thought that they might be dealing with cases of childhood MPD. However, in only a score of instances was the contact of a nature or of sufficient depth to permit pursuit of enough information to ascertain the accuracy of the diagnosis and the characteristics of the treatment process, if any. For example, a perceptive classroom teacher called to discuss how to arrange the assessment of a youngster who showed signs of MPD. The conversation focused primarily on connecting the teacher to authorities in her own area; I avoided all pressures to make a diagnosis over the telephone.

On the basis of approximately 20 colleagues' experiences, the following observations on treatment of childhood MPD are offered. When the treatment situation is controlled, protective, and active and intervenes with the individuals involved, the family, the schools, and so on, it is hard to keep these patients divided. They rapidly recover. When these conditions do not prevail, the patients do not prosper. Their use of dissociative defenses is reinforced and facilitated. Consequently, personalities become more entrenched and may begin to elaborate their identities, and new personalities form in response to new traumata, stresses, and normative developmental conflicts and crises. It is probably impossible to treat an MPD child who is unprotected and/or still suffering abuse. The dissociative defenses offer more relief than anything the therapist can offer.

Some examples may illustrate these issues. A therapist did not believe, in good conscience, that he had sufficient evidence to report child abuse or to confront the parents, even though two children in the family showed signs of MPD. He struggled on with traditional child therapy methods, and neither child improved. Another therapist reported suspected abuse in a case of childhood MPD, but the investigation led to no confirmation of abuse. The child remained within the family, who refused family therapy or treatment of anyone but the child, and the child deteriorated. Another therapist knew of and reported the abuse of a childhood MPD youngster but could not bring himself to recommend removal of the child from the home because he feared the child's mother would commit suicide if this occurred. The child did not improve. In another example, a team of therapists and child protective workers removed an MPD child from an abusive home. She was placed in an abusive foster home, removed, placed in an institution, and then returned to another foster case situation that miscarried, and this cycle was repeated. Despite their best efforts, the child was repeatedly retraumatized and developed more than 25 alter personalities before her 10th birthday. A final example depicts a miscarriage of treatment due to therapist rigidity. A therapist insisted on treating an MPD child with very conservative child analytic techniques, restricting herself largely to interpretive interventions. She did not heed a consultant's advice to inform herself about MPD, to be more active, or to at least consult a more senior and/or certified child analyst as to whether her treatment approach was appropriate for this particular patient. Three years later, she informed the consultant that the patient's family had removed her from treatment after two years of unproductive therapy.

In sum, these anecdotal materials are consistent with the findings in the published literature.

SUGGESTED THERAPEUTIC APPROACHES

The following approaches are derived from clinical experience. Taken as a whole, they invite comparison with Braun's schematization of the treatment of the adult patient (see Chapter 1). The major differences are related to 1) the vulnerable and dependent situation of the MPD child; 2) the less complexity of child MPD patients relative to adult MPD patients; and 3) the MPD child's less intense investment in retaining separate personalities, once they know help is available. Consequently, there is a greater emphasis on clearing the way and providing a favorable environment for the child's resumption of normal growth and development than there is on the intricacies of relating to the alter personalities. The steps outlined below do not form a neat sequence. In clinical practice, they usually overlap, and all remain ongoing once initiated. In some cases, many steps occur simultaneously and are completed over very brief periods of time. This set of steps does not include the development of trust, with which many strategies begin. My experience has been that the first apparent trust is really based on a stance of desparate hope, a "flight into trust," and/or a dissociatively influenced overpositive valuation of the therapist. Genuine trust develops slowly and gradually. Here it is regarded as an ongoing development that progresses slowly as the steps are negotiated.

Step 1 involves preparing oneself for conducting all interventions along the principle, *primum non nocere*, or "First, do no harm." Although most of the cases reported in the literature reached their therapists with much already known, and the therapists had a mandate to treat, in clinical practice one cannot assume this will be the case. When the clinician begins to suspect he is dealing with childhood MPD, he or she must realize that a difficult area is being entered, in which false steps may be difficult to retrieve and decisions may be hard to make but must be reached. If the therapist is unfamiliar with MPD or the normative childhood phenomena with which childhood MPD might be confused, is not clear about his or her legal obligations with respect to reporting suspected child abuse, or is unsure about the impacts of the interventions he or she plans upon possible court proceedings, the therapist must seek out information and/or obtain consultation. If the therapist is unprepared to deal with or provide the wide number and variety of interventions that may prove necessary, he or she must ascertain what resources are available, through agencies or via the collaboration of colleagues. The sequence of events that may come to pass should be anticipated, and nothing done to jeopardize a fair and felicitous outcome. If there is no doubt about the diagnosis from first contact, treatment must be supportive until the patient's safety is ensured. These concerns may appear overstated, but many psychiatrists who find themselves in the midst of such situations are relative neophytes in many of the areas of knowledge and types of procedures with which they must contend.

Under the aegis of such concerns, Step 2, assessment and documentation, has of course already been set in progress. In this process, the therapist must evaluate the patient and the patient's family and/or caretakers. It is useful to establish from the first that the acquisition of all information is imperative and to obtain necessary releases. The use of screening questions with ancillary sources may be helpful. Fagan and McMahon's questions were created with such applications in mind (1984). Leading questions should be avoided as long as possible, but at times they are inevitable. Abused children often learn to scan adults perceptively and may respond as they think the interviewer wishes them to. They have learned that displeasing an adult may be followed by severe consequences. Conversely, many abused children are threatened with punishment if they reveal their experiences, and thus they withhold relevant data. Still others have become accustomed to not being believed and for that reason do not reveal critical materials to the therapist (Goodwin 1985). However useful in treatment, hypnosis should be used with caution during the assessment process. If hypnosis is to be used and there is reason to believe legal proceedings may be necessary, it may prove prudent to document in detail what is discovered prior to hypnosis and to videotape the hypnotic assessment. Forensic guidelines should be followed in case it becomes necessary to use the assessment as evidence in legal proceedings. Many lawyers and judges hold serious reservations about information elicited under hypnosis, and the admissibility of hypnotically retrieved information varies widely in different jurisdictions (Tuite et al. 1986). It is useful to devote enough time to assessing the child's parents that they feel treated with respect and concern. In such a context, it becomes possible to share concerns about abuse and explore what steps must be taken.

After the diagnosis has been established and the family constellation and/or living situation has been assessed, Step 3 entails obtaining control over the situation and establishing the protection of the patient and the treatment. This step also involves attempting to build a therapeutic alliance with the patient's parents and/or caretakers, even if there are adversarial aspects to the situation. If the patient is in danger from self-inflicted harm, a structured environment may be necessary. If intrafamilial abuse exists, it must be reported and the appropriate agencies enlisted to support (or even mandate) treatment and initiate either a supervision of the family or placement of the child. If the child is placed, the safety of the placement must be ensured. If the abuser does not reside with the family, steps must be undertaken to interdict the abuser's access to the child. Through all such efforts, the therapist must try to minimize the secondary traumatization that often accompanies the reporting of abuse and the events that follow in its wake. Again, it is impossible and probably unwise to treat an MPD child still suffering from or unprotected from abuse in any manner other than supportively. The dissociative barriers are some protection to the child. In the unlikely event they were eroded while the child was at risk, the formation of other alternate personalities or overt self-destructive acts are likely outcomes. The former outcome has been documented. The child's social and academic safety must be assured. Although some teachers are understanding and supportive, this is not invariably the case. Furthermore, some children have manifestations that make them unmanageable or expose them to interpersonal risks with long-term deleterious consequences. A period of home tutoring may be preferable to the child's spending several hours a day experiencing rejection, humiliation, and estrangement from his or her peers. This is especially crucial in small town situations. Another aspect of control and protection involves ensuring the establishment of appropriate therapies for others concerned with the case, establishing sanction for ongoing communications between and among all involved therapists, and pacing the child's treatment with the progress of the other therapies.

Step 4 involves the introduction of an active stance into the therapy sessions. The therapist should not hesitate to structure the treatment, to educate patients about their circumstances and their misconceptions about them; to pursue and bring into the therapy, albeit gently, any personalities who wish to evade treatment; and to begin, with kindness and tact, the recollection of events that the patient would prefer to leave banished from available memory. Specific techniques to bring about these objectives, such as play therapy and/or hypnosis, may be introduced.

As a consequence of this stance, the therapist helps the patient achieve Step 5, a preliminary comprehension of his or her circumstances. This must occur at least in the presenting personality. Ideally, this will occur in the other personalities as well. Only when the youngster has an age-appropriate understanding of why he or she is in treatment can participation in Step 6, forming a therapeutic alliance, be permitted. When the child is old enough to grasp the fact of his or her partnership in the treatment, the child often experiences a profound sense of incipient mastery over previously overwhelming processes and finds self-esteem increasing as he or she encounters and deals with the processes.

Step 7 involves an exploration of the patient's consciously available history, experiences, feelings, and perceptions, in all accessible and available personalities, in an atmosphere of empathic acceptance. Efforts may be made to recover repressed material via play techniques and hypnosis. In the process, the child is reeducated with respect to cognitive, affective, communicative, and moral distortions to which he or she has been exposed and is exculpated, at least intellectually, from irrational attributions of blame and sinister motivations. Commonly, MPD children have been told or have come to believe that they are at fault for whatever has befallen them. For example, a girl was assigned a chore inappropriate for someone so young and failed to complete it to her mother's satisfaction. The mother beat her mercilessly "because she was so bad." The little girl accepted this mislabeling, which had to be corrected. When this type of exploration, which may occur quite rapidly, precedes abreaction of traumata, rerepression is less likely. However, rerepression remains common. It is worth noting that some MPD children (and adults) spontaneously abreact and/or collapse their separateness during the process of exploration. When separateness is ceded in this fashion, the issues of the previously separate personalities should not be presumed to be resolved. They will require standard therapeutic efforts. For example, my patient Tommy, whom I mentioned earlier, rapidly fused two female personalities without prior therapeutic work. It was only long after integration that Tommy returned to the problem of confused sexual identity and resolved it satisfactorily. He has gone on to establish a very normal and strong male identity. Another patient, Bobby, became eager to integrate before he was willing to retain recollection of his traumatization. He integrated and rerepressed the historical materials, which were managed subsequently. As this stage gains momentum, it usually becomes possible to discover and bring into the treatment previous oppositional, reluctant, and evasive alters.

Step 8, if it has not occurred admixed with previous steps, is abreaction. Simple intellectual recall or abreaction without an intellectual framework and perspective (see Chapter 1) does not suffice. Here there is a firm place for the use of evocative play therapy, imagery, and hypnotic techniques. Alternate personalities may share these experiences. If they do not, the personalities who are unfamiliar with the abreacted events may have to face them later as fusion proceeds. In younger patients, the abreactive process is rarely contained within the therapy hour. The patient's caretakers must be made aware that prolonged periods of crying and strong feelings are part of the therapeutic process. They must be educated not to stifle the process and inadvertently encourage rerepression. The author has found it productive to return to traumatic material instead of trusting that a single abreactive effort will suffice.

Step 9 entails working through and grief work. The child must explore different facets of what has occurred and often mourns the loss of defensive idealizations, overpositive perceptions of their abusers, shorn of the negative and repressed aspects. The personalities who do not spontaneously fuse must share feelings with one another. A failure to do these things may leave intact dissociatively split object perceptions, which superficially resemble borderline structures. This step also serves to guard against massive rerepression. Some rerepression appears inevitable. In most patients, the memories gradually are retrieved and processed in the postfusion therapy.

By this point, usually much of Step 10, reconciliation of the personalities, has occurred. They have worked together and communicated with and overheard one another throughout the therapy and now the *raison d'être* for their separateness has been ablated. At this point, most child MPD patients do not appear to be strongly motivated to retain the separateness. Instead, they want to join and be normal. By delaying a formal approach to fusion/integration until this point, there usually is minimal resistance. Differences among the personalities are addressed, such as divergent coping styles, unique characteristics, and ages. Age progression fantasies, usually involving imagery and often facilitated by hypnosis, are quite helpful. Personalities begin to feel more alike or are encouraged to communicate, share time together, and so on. By this process of sharing, reconciling, and minimizing differences prior to pressing for fusion, issues of rivalry and/or enmity among the personalities or fretting, "Who will survive?" rarely are encountered. The style of the therapy and the sequence of interventions postpones such matters until they have ceased to have psychological importance. The personalities in children who have MPD, as noted above, rarely become narcissistically invested in separateness to any significant extent prior to early adolescence.

Reconciliation is followed by Step 11, integration, which technically consists of all steps that erode separateness prior to fusion; fusion; and all postfusion efforts to resolve residual tendencies to use dissociative defenses or the formation of alter personalities as a means of solving problems or managing subsequent traumata or dysphoria. Although there is a place for other resolutions (such as negotiated cooperation among alternate personalities or the subsiding of all personalities but one while the rest remain separate but quiescent) in adult patients, this is not acceptable in the treatment of children. Youngsters have many crucial developmental phases yet to negotiate and should be allowed to do so in as normal a manner as possible. In these younger patients, it appears that abreaction and fusion often coincide (Fagan and McMahon 1984). When this does not occur, imagery techniques (Braun 1983, 1984; Kluft 1982, 1984a,

1985a, 1985b) may be effective. In the case reported by Weiss (1985), it is not clear whether integration was pursued after disquieting symptoms subsided. In general, it is not safe to assume that the absence of apparent symptoms indicates that MPD has been treated definitively. It is prudent to search out signs of residual separateness during follow-up session (Kluft 1984b, 1985d).

Postintegration treatment is Step 12. It is crucial to realize that integration, although dramatic, is only one aspect of the overall therapy. Postintegration treatment may be more prolonged than the treatment that facilitated integration. Clinicians should bear in mind that the most challenging aspect of treating childhood MPD lies in stabilizing the child's gains, making sure the normative processes of growth and development are resumed. It is essential to ensure that those who will continue to be involved in the child's life have made stable constructive changes in any of their pathological behavioral patterns and communicative styles. It is crucial that the therapist remain available for ongoing consultation with the institutions that influence the youngster's life.

Step 13 is defined as a periodic follow-up of the childhood MPD patient into late adolescence. My experience is that by doing this, the therapist is often in a position to assist both the child, the parents or caretakers, and the child's other siblings to address incipient problems before they become critical.

The treatment plan delineated in these 13 steps presents my synthesis of currently available publications, my experiences, and colleagues' anecdotal materials. I have shared this treatment plan with several therapists working with cases of childhood MPD. They have reported that it is useful in their hands and that patients they have treated in this manner have done well. However, the study of childhood MPD is just beginning. This treatment plan must be regarded as provisional until it has been critically assessed objectively by other workers, and has been compared, under appropriately controlled circumstances, to other therapeutic approaches as they become available.

REFERENCES

Albini TK, Schwartz TP: Normal and pathological dissociations in young children, Dissociative Disorders 1985: Proceedings of the

Second International Conference on Multiple Personality/Dissociative States. Edited by Braun BG. Chicago, Rush University, 1985

American Psychiatric Association: Diagnostic and Statistical Manual of Mental Disorders (Third Edition). Washington, DC, American Psychiatric Association, 1980

Bliss EL: Multiple personalities, related disorders, and hypnosis. Am J Clin Hypn 26:114–123, 1983

Bliss EL: Spontaneous self-hypnosis in multiple personality disorder. Psychiatr Clin North Am 7:135–148, 1984a

Bliss EL: Hysteria and hypnosis. J Nerv Ment Dis 172:203–206, 1984b

Boor M, Coons PM: A comprehensive bibliography of literature pertaining to multiple personality. Psychol Rep 53:295–310, 1983

Bowers MK, Brecher-Marer S, Newton BW, et al: Therapy of multiple personality. Int J Clin Exp Hypn 19:57–65, 1971

Braun BG: Hypnosis for multiple personalities, in Clinical Hypnosis in Medicine. Edited by Wain HJ. Chicago, Year Book Publishers, 1980

Braun BG: Neurophysiologic changes in multiple personality due to integration: a preliminary report. Am J Clin Hypn 26:84–92, 1983

Braun BG: Use of hypnosis with multiple personality. Psychiatric Annals 14:34–40, 1984

Braun BG: The transgenerational incidence of dissociation and multiple personality disorder: a preliminary report, in Childhood Antecedents of Multiple Personality. Edited by Kluft RP. Washington, DC, American Psychiatric Press, 1985

Braun BG, Sachs RG: The development of multiple personality disorder: predisposing, precipitating, and perpetuating factors, in Childhood Antecedents of Multiple Personality. Edited by Kluft RP. Washington, DC, American Psychiatric Press, 1985

Coons PM: Children of parents with multiple personality disorder, in Childhood Antecedents of Multiple Personality. Edited by Kluft RP. Washington, DC, American Psychiatric Press, 1985

Damgaard J, Van Benschoten S, Fagan J: An updated bibliography of literature pertaining to multiple personality. Psychol Rep 57: 131–137, 1985

Despine P: De l'emploi du magnetisme animal et des eaux minerales dans le traitement des maladies nerveuses, suivi d'une observation tres curieuse de guerison de neuropathie. Paris, Germer, Bailliere, 1840

de Vito RA: Explorations into the phenomenology, etiology, and treatment of multiple personality disorder (MPD), in Dissociative Disorders 1984: Proceedings of the First International Conference on Multiple Personality/Dissociative States. Edited by Braun BG. Chicago, Rush University, 1984

Ellenberger HF: The Discovery of the Unconscious. New York, Basic Books, 1970

Elliott D: State intervention and childhood multiple personality disorder. Journal of Psychiatry and the Law 10:441–456, 1982

Fagan J, McMahon PP: Incipient multiple personality in children: four cases. J Nerv Ment Dis 172:26–36, 1984

Goodwin J: Credibility problems in multiple personality disorder patients and abused children, in Childhood Antecedents of Multiple Personality. Edited by Kluft RP. Washington, DC, American Psychiatric Press, 1985

Greaves GB: Multiple personality: 165 years after Mary Reynolds. J Nerv Ment Dis 168:577–596, 1980

Horevitz RP, Braun BG: Are multiple personalities borderline? in Symposium on Multiple Personality. Edited by Braun BG. Psychiatr Clin North Am 7:69–87, 1984

Kluft RP: Varieties of hypnotic interventions in the treatment of multiple personality disorder. Am J Clin Hypn 24:230–240, 1982

Kluft RP: Multiple personality in childhood, in Symposium on Multiple Personality. Edited by Braun BG. Psychiatr Clin North Am 7:121–134, 1984a

Kluft RP: Treatment of multiple personality disorder: a study of 33 cases, in Symposium on Multiple Personality. Edited by Braun BG. Psychiatr Clin North Am 7:9–29, 1984b

Kluft RP: Childhood multiple personality disorder, in Childhood Antecedents of Multiple Personality. Edited by Kluft RP, Washington, DC, American Psychiatric Press, 1985a

Kluft RP: Hypnotherapy of childhood multiple personality disorder. Am J Clin Hypn 27:201–210, 1985b

Kluft RP: The treatment of multiple personality disorder: current concepts, in Directions in Psychiatry (Volume 5). Edited by Flach FF. New York, Hatherleigh, 1985c

Kluft RP: Using hypnotic inquiry protocols to monitor treatment progress and stability in multiple personality disorder. Am J Clin Hypn 28:63–75, 1985d

Kluft RP, Braun BG, Sachs RG: Multiple personality, intrafamilial abuse, and family psychiatry. International Journal of Family Psychiatry 5:283–301, 1984

Lipman LS: Hypnotizability and multiple personality. Presented at the annual meeting of the American Psychiatric Association, Dallas, 1985

Lipman LS, Braun BG, Frischholz EJ: Hypnotizability and multiple personality disorder: Part 1, Overall hypnotic responsivity, in Dissociative States 1984: Proceedings of the First International Conference on Multiple Personality/Dissociative States. Edited by Braun BG. Chicago, Rush University, 1984

Marmer SS: Psychoanalysis of multiple personality. Int J Psychoanal 61:439–459, 1980

Orne MT: The use and misuse of hypnosis in court. Int J Clin Exp Hypn 27:311–341, 1979

Putnam FW, Guroff JJ, Silberman EK, et al: The clinical phenomenology of multiple personality disorder: 100 recent cases. J Clin Psychiatry 47:285–293, 1986

Schultz, RK, Braun BG, Kluft RP: Creativity and the imaginary companion phenomenon: prevalence and phenomenology in MPD, in Dissociative States 1985: Proceedings of the Second International Conference on Multiple Personality/Dissociative States. Edited by Braun BG. Chicago, Rush University, 1985

Spiegel H, Spiegel D: Trance and Treatment. New York, Basic Books, 1978

Summit RC: The child abuse accommodation syndrome. J Child Abuse Negl 7:177–193, 1983

Tuite P, Braun BG, Frischholz E: Hypnosis and eyewitness testimony. Psychiatric Annals 16:91–95, 1986

Weiss M, Sutton PJ, Utecht AJ: Multiple personality in a 10-year-old girl. J Am Acad Child Psychiatry 24:495–501, 1985

Wilbur CB: Multiple personality and child abuse, in Symposium on Multiple Personality. Edited by Braun BG. Psychiatr Clin North Am 7:3–8, 1984

5

The Dilemma of Drug Therapy for Multiple Personality Disorder

Robert Barkin, M.B.A., Pharm.D.
Bennett G. Braun, M.D.
Richard P. Kluft, M.D.

5

The Dilemma of Drug Therapy for Multiple Personality Disorder

Clinicians have become accustomed to being able to predict the therapeutic, adverse, and side effects of prescription drugs with some degree of certainty. In most patient populations, such predictability is possible and assumed and guides our practice. However, this degree of certainty is the exception rather than the rule when we administer to or prescribe drug therapy for patients with multiple personality disorder (MPD). These individuals do not respond to drugs in a consistent and predictable manner. Different personalities in the same body may respond differently to a given dose of the same medication.

Multiple personality disorder is associated with significant differences and changes across personalities that may be psychological (Brandsma and Ludwig 1974; Larmore et al. 1977), psychophysiological (Bliss 1980; Braun 1983b; Braun and Braun 1979; Brende 1984; Putnam 1983, 1984b), and/or neurophysiological (Braun 1983a). All such differences and changes may depend on which personality has executive control of the body at the time the change occurs. Other personalities of the MPD patient may not demonstrate parallel or other changes during the same period.

Psychophysiological differences (Braun 1983b; Putnam 1984b)

described across personalities include different handedness, accelerated healing processes, and variable medication responses (Barkin et al. 1985; Braun 1983b). Braun (1983b) also described different allergic responses, dermatologic reactions (specific soaps, keratinized plaque, skin spotting, pain and redness), various autonomic nervous system effects (vascular changes, headaches, shifts in heart rate, differential galvanic skin responses), and the ability to control pain by dissociation. Case reports of central nervous system changes in MPD patients clearly include psychogenic epilepsy, tonic-clonic variety, electroencephalogram abnormalities, and neurophysiological changes (Braun 1983a; Putnam 1984b).

Drug effects and reactions are not uniform in their healing effects on persons (Hahn et al. 1986). Perhaps the psychophysiologic phenomena of MPD contribute to the unpredictability in MPD patients' responses to medication (Braun 1984b; Kluft 1984a; Putnam 1984b).

In this chapter, the therapeutic categories of drugs that act on the central nervous system and their expected effects on the general patient population are described, and then each category's effects on MPD patients are described. Generic drug names are used in the discussion of psychotherapeutic agents. At the end of the chapter is an appendix containing some of the more frequently encountered generic and trade names. More comprehensive treatment of basic pharmacology and clinical drug use is offered in Goodman and Gilman's (1985) *The Pharmacologic Basis of Therapeutics*, Schatzberg and Cole's (1986) *Clinical Guide to Psychopharmacology*, and Hahn et al.'s (1986) *Pharmacology in Nursing*.

General agreement exists among clinicians who have significant experience in treating MPD patients that intervention with psychiatric drug therapy may be necessary to relieve some intense specific symptoms. They concur that such prescription use must be prudent and judicious because of the potential for variations in drug response and differences in the adverse effect and side effect profiles among and across the separate personalities (Kluft 1984). Considerations were summarized by Kluft (1984a):

Neither automatically denying nor readily acceding to the patient's requests for relief is reasonable. Several questions must be raised: 1) Is the distress part of a medication-responsive syndrome? 2) If the answer to 1) is yes, is it of sufficient clinical importance to outweigh possible adverse impacts of prescription? If the answer to 1) is no, whom would the drug treat (the physician's need to "do something," an anxious third party, etc.)? 3) Is there a non-pharmacological intervention which might prove effective instead? 4) Does the overall management require an intervention which the psychiatrist realizes is non-specific, but feels is essential? 5) What is the patient's "track record" in response to interventions similar to the one which is planned? 6) Weighing all considerations, do the potential benefits outweigh the potential risks? Medication abuse and ingestions with prescribed drugs are common risks. (p. 53)

In this chapter we attempt to distill anecdotal experience that reflects our personal therapeutic experience and that expressed by our respective patient populations. This information is presented in an area in which there is a paucity of well-controlled studies.

In working with these patients, the clinician may be prescribing drugs approved by the Food and Drug Administration (FDA), but the indication for which the clinician is using the drugs may not be among those with FDA approval. Prudent clinical judgment necessitates informing the patient of any use of a drug that is a departure from FDA-approved uses. Informed consent is important when nontraditional forms of drug therapy are used as treatment modalities. In Chapter 1 of this book, Braun describes a therapeutic contracting technique. These therapeutic contracts are reviewed with all interested personalities. Those personalities unable to verbally express their acceptance and understanding of the contract may express themselves in agreement by idiomotor signal movements (see Chapter 1). Putnam (1984a) in consultation with the Bioethics Committee of the National Institute of Mental Health suggested that only one signature is needed for informed consent after the information is explained to a given personality and all of those willing to participate.

The variable responses by MPD patients to medication may be more easily understood in view of the implications of the aforementioned psychophysiologic phenomena: The patient suffering from MPD has several patterns of psychophysiological organization, more or less associated with the several personalities, and depending on which personality or personalities are in control, a uniform stimulus or pharmacologic agent may be processed differently and therefore have a different effect.

Care must be taken in the use of medication with MPD patients. They are more prone to both accidental (e.g., several personalities taking a medicine not knowing that others already had taken it) overdose and intentional overdose as suicide and "internal homicide" attempts. They also are prone to physical and psychological addictions.

Generally, if one of the personalities of an MPD patient is a former drug abuser, this personality may be so protective or guarded as to reject all of a clinician's attempts at therapeutic medication. This is done out of fear of relapsing into chemical dependence. In addition, the patient may view the prescription of medication as an act to threaten and overthrow a drug-free state.

ANXIOLYTIC AGENTS

Use of Anxiolytics in General Patient Populations

Anxiolytic drug therapy (benzodiazepines, hydroxyzine, meprobamate) is commonly directed at relief of dysphoria associated with atypical and generalized anxiety states, panic and phobic disorders, agoraphobia, and posttraumatic stress disorder. When coupled with appropriate psychotherapy, anxiolytic drug therapy has predictable outcomes in the general population. Not infrequently it produces relief of persistent anxiety; facilitates management of recognizable stress; and diminishes recurrent distressing dreams, motor tension, autonomic hyperactivity, apprehensive expectation, vigilance and scanning, persistent and irrational fears, and excessive and unreasonable panic.

Meprobamate is one of the oldest of the anxiolytic drugs. The documented side effects of meprobamate include sedation and drowsiness, even in therapeutic dosages. On rare occasions its use is complicated by blood dyscrasias and purpura. Chemical dependency including habituation and physical dependence has been seen with long-term administration. Discontinuance of meprobamate therapy must be gradual in order to avoid a withdrawal syndrome. Paraldehyde, which is even older, has been used as a last resort with mixed results in both the general population and in MPD patients.

The introduction of the benzodiazepines has led to a great reduction in the use of meprobamate. The benzodiazepines as a group have sedative and to a lesser extent mild hypnotic properties. In addition, they possess some central skeletal muscle relaxant activity. They also can produce a degree of chemical dependency. Psychological and physical dependence are liabilities, and withdrawal phenomena may be encountered as well.

The effects from benzodiazepines on the central nervous system include central nervous system depression, in particular within the limbic system area. Benzodiazepines are thought to potentiate the effects of gamma-aminobutyric acid within the central nervous system. These actions may contribute to the anxiolytic effects of the benzodiazepines. The side effects or adverse effects most frequently reported in the general population are ataxia, drowsiness, and sedation. The modulation of such effects may be dose related in some patients. Additive central nervous system depressant effects are seen when these agents are administered concurrently with other central nervous system depressing drugs. Chemical dependency may develop. Withdrawal symptoms are likely to arise following the abrupt discontinuation of long-term, high-dose regimens. Benzodiazepines with a long half-life usually have desmethyldiazepam as an intermediate metabolite. The onset of withdrawal phenomena may be initially delayed, but ultimately prolonged in duration because of the self-tapering effect of the long half-life. The withdrawal symptoms may not occur until 7 to 10 days following discontinuation of therapy. This is not generally seen with those benzodiazepines lacking desmethyldiazepam as an intermediate metabolite, such as alprazolam, lorazepam, and oxazepam. Withdrawal phenomena from these benzodiazepines occur within two days of discontinuing the therapy.

Alprazolam, an intermediate-acting benzodiazepine, is not an antidepressant (polycyclic or monoamine oxidase inhibitor) but is indicated for depression secondary to anxiety. It is generally well accepted by MPD patients. Its half-life ranges from 12 to 15 hours. It also shows dependency and withdrawal problems when used in higher doses over prolonged time periods.

Effects of Anxiolytics on Multiple Personality Disorder Patients

Multiple personality disorder patients generally experience an irregular, unpredictable anxiolytic drug impact on their personality systems. If the anxiety level is high across all the personalities or predominates in a personality who is critical to daily functioning, then circumspect benzodiazepine use may be justified. Use of benzodiazepines for periods of time may also be indicated 1) to calm the overall patient or particular personalities during initial treatment periods, 2) to diminish the anxiety that emerges in the course of intense treatment periods, 3) to palliate anxiety and stress-mediated phenomena associated with the integration process, 4) to stabilize the patient while developing and maturing nondissociative coping mechanisms that had been nonexistent or immature, and 5) to relieve any prolonged anxiety during the postintegration periods in responsible and accountable patients.

Besides providing the expected and desired results, anxiolytic drugs have some unpredictable and inconsistent effects on MPD patients. Instances have been noted in which, for example, 5 mg of diazepam made one personality of a patient sedated, whereas a 200 mg self-administered dose taken by a different personality of the same patient had little effect on the patient's abilities to remain alert. Other outcomes of benzodiazepine therapy reported anecdotally are no effect at all among adult personalities, paradoxical activation or disinhibition of aggression, decrease in shaking and fears, drowsiness, dysphoria, and racing thoughts. Among child personalities within the system the following effects were reported: passing out, drowsiness, staggering gait, and paradoxical fears. Hyperactive child personalities report no effect.

The characteristic response profile of the personality who maintains executive control of the body is a major determinant of the impact of the anxiolytic medication. One personality may experience the predictable effects seen in the general population, but the protective or aggressive personalities may not. In other words, in addition to the different personalities' having various sensitivities to a given dose of medication, an identical dose may also elicit different qualitative responses. For example, in one patient meprobamate sedated some protector personalities but brought to the surface or unleashed overt hostile manifestations in other personalities within the system. A younger personality demonstrated hyperactivity, an increased level of energy, and increased disorganization of thought. A related drug, carisprodol, produced confusion and racing thoughts in adult personalities, but in a younger personality within the same body it produced sleep, relaxation, and decreased energy.

SEDATIVE/HYPNOTICS

Use of Sedative/Hypnotics in General Patient Populations

Drugs within this class include benzodiazepines and the non-benzodiazepines. The benzodiazepines classified as sedative/hypnotics include triazolam, temazepam, flurazepam, and lorazepam. They are indicated for short-term management of insomnia characterized by difficulty in falling or staying asleep, frequent nocturnal and/or early morning awakening, or insomnia secondary to anxiety or transient situational stresses. The nonbenzodiazepine sedative/hypnotics include barbiturates, chloral hydrate, ethchlorvynol, glutethimide, methaqualone, methyprylon, and paraldehyde. In the general population, patients who take barbiturates and other nonbenzodiazepine sedative/hypnotics are subject to chemical dependence and intoxication.

Physiological as well as psychological dependence may occur. Withdrawal symptoms may emerge with glutethimide, methyprylon, ethchlorvynol, and methaqualone. Used in the general population, chloral hydrate is a relatively safe hypnotic with an onset of approximately 30 to 60 minutes. It causes a small reduction in rapid eye movement sleep, is irritating to the gastrointestinal tract, and has an objectionable taste. Paraldehyde produces sleep in approximately 15 minutes; it has some central nervous system depressant activity resembling that of alcohol, chloral hydrate, and barbiturates. Paraldehyde has a strong odor and disagreeable taste, which limits its use, especially in outpatient populations. Glutethimide is highly subject to abuse and chemical dependence and has its own withdrawal symptoms. Chronic use has lead to toxicity, convulsions and hyperpyrexia, and an extreme anticholinergic effect. The drug is subject to abuse when used alone or in combination with other drugs (for example, codeine). Methyprylon in the general population resembles the rapid-acting barbiturates such as secobarbital in both onset and duration of action. Adverse and side effects generally reported are hangover, skin rashes, and some degree of chemical dependence. Ethchlorvynol has an onset of approximately 30 minutes after absorption from the gastrointestinal tract. Its adverse and side effects include ataxia, facial numbness and tingling, and hypotension. This drug is subject to a high degree of psychological dependence, and physical dependence can occur. Its use is substantially limited to less than a week without further evaluation. Methaqualone is a drug that has experienced substantial abuse and is no longer available in the United States as a prescription drug. Patients often describe mini-seizures that may occur prior to onset of sleep, and daytime hangover is common. In addition, physical dependence and tolerance occur.

Effects of Sedative/Hypnotics on Multiple Personality Disorder Patients

Attempts to use hypnotics in MPD patients have had mixed outcomes. There are anecdotal reports describing an absence of effects or sedation, ataxia, and unleashed disinhibition among different personalities within the same system. The results obtained are a function of the differential effects upon the several personalities. Sedative hypnotics may inhibit or sedate the presenting personality and may allow for ascendency of other personalities, thereby yielding unexpected behavior including disinhibition of aggression. Because accommodation rapidly occurs, the alternation of two or more sedative/hypnotic agents over short periods may be beneficial in some MPD patients who have insomnia. Psychotherapy is necessary to uncover the reasons for insomnia (for example, somatic memory or somatization) because often the patient uses the sedative/hypnotic medication as a form of chemical dissociation.

The benzodiazepine sedative/hypnotics generally have had favorable results in MPD patients. Predictable effects were seen with triazolam and temazepam. To date, this has been achieved without causing any daytime sedation or any of the other adverse effects that have been seen in the general population. Triazolam's onset of action is more rapid than the onsets of temazepam and flurazepam. Patients who receive lorazepam for inducing sleep may report a lack of recall of events of the preceding day.

The nonbenzodiazepine sedative/hypnotics are highly subject to abuse and misuse by patients, as are all drugs within this category. Patient automanipulation of dose and/or frequency can produce devastating outcomes. Cautious, highly supervised, infrequent use is the rule with this group of drugs. Barbiturates have a broad range of effects, from no reported effect to induction of sleep with supratherapeutic dosage of rapid-acting barbiturates. Paraldehyde effects within the same system of MPD patients ranged from no effect to sedation, drunken feeling in adult personalities, and hyperactivity or unconsciousness in child personalities. Chloral hydrate had no effect in some personalities and placed others in a state of sleep. Combinations of amobarbital and diazepam in large doses did not induce sleep in some patients within four hours. A host personality may not permit sleep medication to take effect due to a fear of losing control.

Ethchlorvynol has produced central nervous system stimulation and made some personalities feel more in control, which reinforces its abuse potential. Ethinamate, glutethimide, and ethchlorvynol are generally inappropriate hypnotic therapy in MPD patients because of their abuse, toxicity, side/adverse effects profile and their narrow therapeutic to toxic dose range. Benzodiazepines offer a more rational alternative.

Because mixed and inconsistent results are not infrequent, problems of tolerance and abuse are not uncommon. It may be prudent to capitalize on the sedative effects of other drugs that are prescribed to treat concurrent disease states in order to initiate sedation (for example, antihistamines, antidysrhythmics, some antihypertension agents, antiemetics, neuroleptics, and other drugs with anticholinergic or sedative side effects). Drugs that have sedative side/adverse effects may be administered as close to the patient's bedtime as pharmacologically and pharmacokinetically possible.

It is critical to realize that sleep disruption due to interpersonality conflict or the reactivations of repressed dysphoric traumatic material may resist all safe psychopharmacological interventions and all subanesthetic doses. This is why MPD patients abuse/overdose medications to achieve relief. It is preferable to educate the patient and arrive at a compromise regimen that offers a modicum of relief rather than to escalate the hypnotic dosage into unacceptable realms. True sleep deprivation crises are one of the rare indications for a trial course of chlorpromazine of short duration.

NEUROLEPTIC DRUGS

Use of Neuroleptics in General Patient Populations

The major indications for neuroleptics (i.e., antipsychotics and major tranquilizers) include management of some symptoms of the psychotic disorders; antiemesis; motion sickness; intractable hiccoughs; presurgical restlessness and apprehension; organic brain syndrome; alcoholism; Tourette's syndrome; as adjunctive therapy in control of manic episodes; and for psychotic depressive episodes, schizophrenia, behavioral problems, mental deficiency, and the excessive impulsive hyperactivity seen with childhood conduct disorders.

Neuroleptics are prescribed to relieve or reduce delusions, hallucinations, incoherence, loosening of associations, illogical thought, inappropriate affect, grossly disorganized behavior, functional deterioration, catatonia, and paranoid ideation.

In the general population the major adverse or side effects upon the central nervous system include 1) Parkinsonian syndrome, exemplified by rigidity and resting tremor; 2) an acute dystonic reaction, which may be seen at the initiation of therapy when the patients display grimacing of facial features and torticollis; 3) tardive dyskinesia, the involuntary display of oral, facial, lingual, and buccal movements that may appear to be sucking and smacking of the lips (this is occasionally seen with chronic therapy and may persist long after therapy is discontinued); and 4) lethargy and drowsiness. Effects on the cardiovascular system include orthostatic hypotension that may precipitate syncope and reflex tachycardia. Hypotension is an important effect not to be overlooked. Allergic reactions also occur, usually within the first few months of therapy, and include cholestatic jaundice, blood dyscrasia, and eosinophilia. Many forms of dermatitis are seen. They include photosensitivity reactions, requiring the use of sun screening agents. The anticholinergic effects may produce blurred vision, constipation, xerostomia, decreased sweating, and occasionally urinary retention. These drugs produce little chemical dependency; that is, there is no evidence of physical dependence or habituation. However, this safeguard is offset by their ability to cause reversible and irreversible extrapyramidal symptoms.

Effects of Neuroleptics on Multiple Personality Disorder Patients

Within the system of personalities of the MPD patient, the predictable side, therapeutic, or adverse effects of sedation, extrapyramidal symptoms and orthostasis, autonomic effects, antimuscarinic effects, tardive dyskinesia, and cardiovascular problems may be experienced sometimes as a frontal assault directed against a specific personality or personalities. This may attenuate or paralyze that personality or change the personality's position within the system. Reality orientation or the patient's feeling of being in control of himself may be broken, creating disequilibrium. In response to this turmoil, increase in splitting and switching within the system may occur in a misguided effort to cope. A new personality may be created or former ones may reemerge in response to the sense of disorganization and dysphoria experienced by the neuroleptic-treated MPD patient.

Occasionally one or two doses of a neuroleptic are indicated to calm severe agitation when there is a severe situational disruption of the equilibrium of the system or in sleep deprivation crisis. However, extended use of these medications may prove problematic. There are anecdotally reported risks of protectors becoming sedated and of difficulty in controlling hostile behaviors and maintaining control over other disruptive personalities within the system. Patients describe racing thoughts, hyperactivity, hallucinations, paranoid ideation, drug-induced psychosis, and severe headaches in connection with their undergoing neuroleptic therapy. Many patients report creating more personalities as a defense mechanism to cope with what they feel were neuroleptic-induced adverse effects. Instances have been noted in which such reactions have persisted as long as a month following the cessation of medication. Prochlorperazine, however, has been used successfully for its antiemetic effects during short intermittent periods of acute nausea and vomiting.

Pharmacotherapies indicated for the relief of depression include the polycyclic antidepressants (first and second generation), monoamine oxidase inhibitors, and some benzodiazepines. Besides depression, indications for these medications include anorexia nervosa, bulimia, nocturnal enuresis, anxiety and sleep disturbances secondary to depression, chronic pain syndromes, for delay of onset of cluster and migraine headaches, as adjunctive treatment in obstructive sleep apnea, and peptic ulcer disease. Other therapeutic applications include agoraphobia, panic attacks, social phobia, and cocaine withdrawal. Some of these therapeutic indications may exist concurrently with MPD.

Use of Polycyclic Antidepressants in the General Patient Population

In the general population, depressive symptoms that are amenable to relief by polycyclic antidepressants include appetite disturbances, weight loss, sleep disturbances, decreased energy, psychomotor agitation or retardation, diurnal mood variation, and decreased libido. Subjective symptoms including hopelessness, helplessness, loss of self-esteem, and demoralization respond more favorably to psychotherapy. In the general population, polycyclic antidepressants have documented effects on the central nervous system. The nondepressed individual experiences sleepiness, anxiety, and undesirable anticholinergic affects when this type of antidepressant is administered. A depressed patient generally finds mood improvement to occur within two to three weeks following initiation of therapy with the correct medication. High dosages and overdosages of these drugs may produce seizures, arrhythmias, and coma. Cardiovascular effects include orthostatic hypotension and arrhythmias. Tachycardia is seen in response to the hypotension. Interference with atrioventricular conduction, which is described as a quinidine-like affect, is also seen. Autonomic nervous system effects, which include the anticholinergic effects, vary among these drugs. Such effects include dry mouth, blurred vision, constipation, disturbances of accommodation, urinary retention, increased intraocular pressure, paralytic ileus, dilatation of urinary tract, mydriasis, and delayed micturition. Amitriptyline has significant incidence of anticholinergic effects. Other adverse effects include diaphoresis, dizziness and muscle trembling in the elderly, skin rashes, and cholestatic jaundice. In patients with bipolar affective disorders, manic excitation and delirium may be produced by these agents. Doxepin has been described as having more sedative results secondary to the anticholinergic or antihistaminic effects.

Effects of Polycyclic Antidepressants on Multiple Personality Disorder Patients

When the host or a prominent personality alone is depressed, there may be no need for antidepressant therapy. When both the host and other personalities within the system are depressed or when depression is prominent in all the personalities, the appropriate use of prescription antidepressants often results in mood elevation. The polycyclic antidepressant may relieve depression and permit more stability to allow for effective application of psychotherapy of the dissociative disorder. Antidepressant drugs have facilitated therapy in patients who have remained blocked for long periods.

The polycyclic antidepressants have also produced inconsistent results within the MPD patient's personalities. The responses are transient and relief may not be achievable in all personalities within the system.

Monoamine Oxidase Inhibitors in the General Patient Population

In the general population, the effects of monoamine oxidase inhibitors on the central nervous system include alleviation of depression. They may be effective in certain sleep disorders, panic disorders, and narcolepsy. Cardiovascular side effects include postural hypotension. The monoamine oxidase inhibitors interact with other drugs (for example, polycyclic antidepressants, sympathomimetic amines) and with foods containing high tyramine content (such as food requiring an aging process, cheese, beer, and chicken livers). Such interactions may produce hypertensive crises. Additional adverse and side effects include hepatocellular damage, especially with the hydrazine monoamine oxidase inhibitors (isocarboxazid, phenelzine). Excessive central nervous system stimulation has been seen, especially with the nonhydrazine, tranylcypromine. This can result in insomnia and convulsions. Overdosage with these agents may produce agitation, hypotension, headache, hypertension, convulsions, and death.

Effects of Monoamine Oxidase Inhibitors on Multiple Personality Disorder Patients

Within the MPD patient population, the use of monoamine oxidase inhibitors is subject to tyramine sabotage by some personalities in a patient's personality system. One personality intending to punish or frighten another personality may overtly produce a hypertensive crisis by ingesting food with a high tyramine content or use a sympathomimetic drug (amphetamines, anorexients, epinephrine, levodopa, methyldopa). The risk may be offset by their usefulness for depression refractory to all other therapeutic modalities. Besides the hoped-for results within the multiple personality system of MPD patients, some patients report no effects and others experience headache, anxiety attacks, heightened fears, and an increase in depressive symptoms.

ANTIMANIC DRUG THERAPY

Lithium Use in the General Patient Population

Lithium is indicated for the treatment of manic episodes of bipolar affective disorders to diminish the frequency and intensity of manic episodes. Additional uses include increasing neutrophilic leukocytosis in cancer chemotherapy and prophylaxis of cluster migraine headache and cyclical migraine headache.

Primary symptoms for which this therapy may be directed include elevated expansive or irritable moods, increased activity, pressured speech, flight of ideas, racing thoughts, inflated self-esteem, decreased sleep requirements, distractability, and involvement in activities with painful consequences. This is true if the patient is suffering from bipolar disorder but not if the symptoms are due to MPD alone. Instances have been noted in which lithium may facilitate the effects of polycyclic antidepressants. Lithium must be monitored attentively for serum levels to remain within the therapeutic range, and toxicity must be avoided.

Lithium does not produce any psychotherapeutic effects in patients without these disorders. In the general patient population the side and adverse effects include fine hand tremor, metallic taste, vomiting, diarrhea, excessive thirst, and polyuria from therapeutic or elevated serum levels of lithium. Seizures, somnolence, confusion, and psychomotor disturbances are reported. Adverse cardiovascular effects include hypotension and arrhythmia, T-wave inversion, and electrocardiogram changes. Chronic use of lithium can result in enlargement of the thyroid gland and various renal effects.

Effects of Lithium on Multiple Personality Disorder Patients

Many MPD patients have been misdiagnosed as having bipolar disorders, and almost all suffer from headache (Braun 1983b, Braun and Braun 1979). It should also be realized that MPD is a superordinate diagnosis (Putnam et al. 1984) and MPD and bipolar disorders can coexist within the same patient (Kluft 1984a; Coryell 1983).

Clinical experience has shown that in some MPD patients lithium appears to suppress personality switching and may appear to reduce some chaotic episodes, many in association with affective disorders when rapid fluctuations in personality appear. It is important to bear in mind that many MPD patients do not respond to lithium at all and that close scrutiny of some alleged positive responses raised questions as to whether the observed changes were due to lithium or other interventions.

MISCELLANEOUS PRESCRIPTION DRUGS

Narcotic Agonists' Effects on Multiple Personality Disorder Patients

A narcotic agonist may be used for the management of pain, diarrhea, anesthesia, and cough. Variable unpredicted effects are seen within the same system of the MPD patient. In one patient, paragoric, used for diarrhea, produced physical and psychological dependence, and drug-seeking behavior in a child personality. Codeine-containing cough syrups caused one patient to create a new personality to assume the addictive liability; to maintain the balance of the system, the problem personality went through withdrawal and surfaced. Teenage personalities may claim expanded feelings, euphoria, and craving. A personality within a female patient's system developed an "allergic" response to morphine, described as hives and itching, to protect her from further use. Meperidine has effects that range from agitation to a drunken feeling, sedation, and amnesia in the same patient, depending on the emergent personality.

The prescription of pain medication requires considerable care because the MPD patient's pain may be of functional origin. Also, the somatic discomfort associated with past abuse may be reexperienced dissociated from the other aspects of memory (affect and knowledge) (Braun 1985). Such pain responds more to appropriate psychotherapeutic interventions than to analgesic therapy. Although it is critical to offer reasonable analgesia, exploration of the etiology of the pain is additionally critical. Otherwise it may become a resistance to psychotherapy and fixate the therapy on the pain and not the underlying problems. Care must be exercised not to become excessively involved in manipulation of dosages and medications.

Other Prescription Medication

The uses for the medications reported below are not all necessarily FDA approved and thus are "experimental." Before departing from FDA approved indications for an already approved medication, it is recommended that other avenues be exhausted. The patient should be verbally informed, and informed consent should be signed if indicated. We are not recommending non-FDA-approved uses; it is up to the individual clinician to determine the course of his or her treatment.

Carbamazepine, an anticonvulsant structurally similar to tricyclic antidepressants, has been used for short periods to manage patients with chaotic, uncontrolled, rapidly fluctuating dissociation. Although a plausible rationale for the effective use of carbamazepine has been offered by clinicians who refer to the possible connection between MPD patients and seizure disorders (Schenk and Bear 1981), clinical results to date have been inconsistent and/or equivocal. The side and adverse effects include ataxia, drowsiness, diplopia, aplastic anemia, agranulocytosis, Stevens-Johnson syndrome, cardiac toxicity, and hepatitis. Clonazepam is a benzodiazepine anticonvulsant that has had variable reports concerning its application to treatment of psychiatric illness. This drug produces frequent drowsiness and sedation in MPD patients. Use of these drugs for indications beyond those approved by FDA becomes experimental.

Methylphenidate had no effect on the personalities, except those under 12 years old. Other patients given methylphenidate described agitation in some personalities within their system and a calming effect on others.

Some other agents that have been used in MPD patients with mixed results to control extremes in anxiety and hyperactivity include the beta-adrenergic-receptor-blocking drugs and the antihypertensive agent clonidine. Beta-adrenergic-blocking agents, such as propranolol, inhibit the patient's response to adrenergic stimuli through competitive blocking of the beta-adrenergic receptors and decreasing of the sympathetic flow from the central nervous system. Clonidine, an alpha-adrenergic agonist, activates the $alpha_2$-adrenergic receptors within the central nervous system. This causes an inhibition but not a blockade of the sympathetic vasomotor centers. Such usages are experimental.

Anesthesia and neuromuscular blocking agents have variable effects within the same system. Patients frequently describe being awake while under anesthesia and talking coherently with members of the surgical team, while unable to move or feel pain during the surgical procedure. Dental procedures often require excess dosages of anesthetic gases and local anesthetics.

The patient's abuse of drugs by a drug-abusing personality within the MPD system often may be understood as a miscarried attempt to self-medicate depression or agitated states. Drug and alcohol-abusing personalities may offer resistance to therapy through use of drugs.

NONPSYCHOTHERAPEUTIC DRUG USE

Drugs of Potential Abuse

Marijuana effects in the MPD patient range from no effects to the achievable "high," depression, and paranoia. Other effects include nausea and vomiting, fear, and paranoia within the same system. Some MPD patients use LSD and other hallucinogens as a form of chemical dissociation. Many MPD patients report bad trips more often than not.

Cocaine when used by MPD patients may facilitate the ascendance of certain types of personalities. The abuse of amphetamines and cocaine may be used by an MPD patient to camouflage dissociation from other personalities within a system and from society as a whole. Amphetamines cause depression in some personalities and elation in others.

Ethanol and other drugs may have been used by external others in childhood, to induce the MPD patient to perform acts that were socially and morally inappropriate and unacceptable. Under these circumstances, some personality of the MPD in adult life will have a low tolerance to the inebriating effects of alcohol; one drink may cause a patient to openly display a drunken appearance. Conversely, some personalities have a high tolerance for alcohol and retain control and memory despite a large ingestion of alcohol. The social personality or personalities may be prevented from achieving the desired effects of drinking by a controlling protective personality within the system.

Ethanol may be used as a self-administered tranquilizer or as an excuse to cover up and/or deny blackouts by the patient. This denial is both for the patient and to the external world. Ethanol consumption and outcomes are completely unpredictable within individual MPD patient systems. Excessive quantities of alcoholic beverages may often be consumed within a short time period with no appreciable effect on some personalities within the system who can speak, walk, and perform college-level work without displaying that the body is under the influence of alcohol. Other personalities may become severely depressed or inebriated or may slide into unconsciousness. The children of the system may be unconscious after the initial two to three drinks (30 ml of 80 proof ethanol equivalent each). An aggressive, violent, or dependent personality may emerge during drinking episodes as the ethanol acts to stimulate emergence of anger and/or dependency through disinhibition mechanisms. Some personalities within the system may be under a contract not to drink, and some personalities may have disease states for which drinking is discouraged.

Over-the-Counter Medications

Over-the-counter medication dose and response differ with personality. Antacid doses needed to decrease gastric acidity are a function of the personality needing them. Phenylpropanolamine, which is present in many over-the-counter anorexiants (diet aids) and in some cough and cold preparations, had no effect in an anorexic personality and increased the appetite of a bulimic personality.

Braun (1983c) suggested that glutamic acid in doses from 500 mg four times a day to 1000 mg three or four times a day decreases the intensity and frequency of certain types of headaches in MPD patients. This affects only the headaches of excessive thinking and/or switching. It does not stop them altogether.

PHYSIOLOGIC AND DISEASE SYMPTOM INCONSISTENCIES

Disease states in conditions such as asthma, diabetes, milk intolerance and allergic diseases, ulcers, and visual impairments may not be present in all personalities within the same MPD patient (Braun 1983b; Shepard and Braun 1985). It is not uncommon for an MPD patient to have multiple sets of eyeglasses or contact lenses to be used among various personalities within the system for whom those eyeglass prescriptions are specific. Instances have been noted within the same MPD patient where glycosuria may be quantitatively different among personalities, and caution must be exercised in using sliding scale insulin adjustments (Braun 1983a, 1983b).

CONCLUSIONS

We are able to discern from our clinical experience that the patient with MPD is subject to the side- and adverse-effect profile of any drug in any therapeutic category. Various personalities respond differently to the same dose of the specific medication. Therapeutic drug use with this patient group is then further complicated by the unpredictable and often paradoxical effects that may occur in any of the emerging, controlling, or prominent personalities that occupy the body during the time the drug is administered or during the time of its absorption, distribution, metabolism, and elimination. We advocate initiating only the drug therapy that is absolutely required to treat the entire personality system of the patient or most of the predominant personalities of the patient. It is prudent to always initiate therapy with a drug that has the fewest or lowest level of side or adverse effects. The initial dosage should be the lowest possible therapeutic dosage. The dose may be titrated upward to meet the individual patient's needs. The MPD patient on medication must be followed carefully and assessed regularly for the medication's therapeutic impact, side effects, and adverse reactions. Polycyclic antidepressants and monoamine oxidase inhibitors are not to be used to treat reactive depression in one or a few personalities in MPD patients but are useful when the depressive symptomatology is generalized across personalities. Benzodiazepines are used to diminish anxiety and to sedate. Anxiety may lead to rapid switching and thus to unintentional overdoses due to the individual needs of personalities that are not co-conscious. Responses to other medications have not been evaluated adequately to permit us to provide significant clinical insights or other guidelines at this time.

REFERENCES

Barkin RL, Braun BG, Kluft RP: The dilemma of drug therapy for multiple personality disorders, in Dissociative Disorders 1985: Proceedings of the Second International Conference on Multiple Personality/Dissociative States. Edited by Braun BG. Chicago, Rush University, 1985

Bliss EL: Multiple personalities: a report of 14 cases with implications for schizophrenia and hysteria. Arch Gen Psychiatry 37:1388–1400, 1980

Brandsma JM, Ludwig AM: A case of multiple personality: diagnosis and therapy. Int J Clin Exp Hypn 22:216–233, 1974

Braun BG: Neurophysiologic changes in multiple personality due to integration: a preliminary report. Am J Clin Hypn 26:84–92, 1983a

Braun BG: Psychophysiologic phenomena in multiple personality and hypnosis. Am J Clin Hypn 26:124–137, 1983b

Braun BG: Therapies for MPD. Presented at the annual meeting of the American Psychiatric Association, New York, 1983c

Braun BG: Towards a theory of multiple personality and other dissociative phenomena, in Symposium on Multiple Personality. Edited by Braun BG. Psychiatr Clin North Am 7:171–193, 1984

Braun BG: Dissociation: behavior, affect, sensation, knowledge, in Dissociative Disorders 1985: Proceedings of the Second International Conference on Multiple Personality/Dissociative States. Edited by Braun BG. Chicago, Rush University, 1985

Braun BG, Braun RE: Clinical aspects of multiple personality. Presented at a meeting of the American Society of Clinical Hypnosis, San Francisco, November 1979

Brende JO: The psychophysiologic manifestations of dissociations, in Symposium on Multiple Personality. Edited by Braun BG. Psychiatr Clin North Am 7:41–50, 1984

Coryell W: Multiple personality and primary affective disorder. J Nerv Ment Dis 171:388–390, 1983

Goodman LS, Gilman AG: The Pharmacologic Basis for Therapeutics (Seventh Edition). New York, Macmillan, 1985

Hahn AB, Barkin RL, Oestreich S: Pharmacology in Nursing (16th Edition). St. Louis, C.V. Mosby, 1986

Kluft RP: Psychopharmacological approaches to multiple personality. Presented at the annual meeting of the American Psychiatric Association, New York, 1983

Kluft RP: Aspects of the treatment of multiple personality disorder. Psychiatric Annals 14:51–55, 1984a

Kluft RP: Treatment of multiple personality disorder, in Symposium on Multiple Personality. Edited by Braun BG. Psychiatr Clin North Am 7:31–40, 1984b

Larmore K, Ludwig AM, Cain RL: Multiple personality: an objective case study. Br J Psychiatry 131:35–40, 1977

Putnam FW: Evoked potentials in multiple personality disorder. Presented at the annual meeting of the American Psychiatric Association, New York, 1983

Putnam FW: The study of multiple personality disorder: general strategies and practical considerations. Psychiatric Annals 14:58–61, 1984a

Putnam FW: The psychophysiologic investigation of multiple personality disorder, in Symposium on Multiple Personality. Edited by Braun BG. Psychiatr Clin North Am 7:31–40, 1984b

Putnam FW, Lowenstein RJ, Silberman EK, et al: Multiple personality disorder in a hospital setting. J Clin Psychiatry 45:172–175, 1984

Schatzberg AF, Cole JO: Clinical Guide to Psychopharmacology. Washington, DC, American Psychiatric Press, 1986

Schenk L, Bear D: Multiple personality and related dissociative phenomena in patients with temporal lobe epilepsy. Am J Psychiatry 138:1311–1316, 1981

Shepard KR, Braun BG: Visual changes in the multiple personality, in Dissociative Disorders 1985: Proceedings of the Second International Conference on Multiple Personality/Dissociative States. Edited by Braun BG. Chicago, Rush University, 1985

APPENDIX

DRUG NAMES DESCRIBED AS GENERIC (TRADE NAMES)

Anxiolytics

Long-acting benzodiazepines
  Chlordiazepoxide (Librium, others)
  Chlorazepate (Tranxene)
  Diazepam (Valium, others)
  Halazepam (Paxipam)
  Prazepam (Centrax)
Short- to intermediate-acting benzodiazepines
  Alprazolam (Xanax)
  Lorazepam (Ativan)
  Oxazepam (Serax)
Other anxiolytics
  Meprobamate (Equanil, Miltown)
  Meprobamate with benzactine (Deprol)
  Chlormezanone (Trancopal)
  Hydroxyzine (Vistaril, Atarax)

Sedative/Hypnotics

Chloral hydrate (Noctec)
Glutethimide (Doriden)
Methyprylon (Noludar)

Ethchlorvynol (Placidyl)
Ethinamate (Valmid)
Benzodiazepines
    Flurazepam (Dalmane)
    Temazepam (Restoril)
    Triazolam (Halcion)

Antidepressants

Polycyclic antidepressants
    Tertiary amines
        Amitriptyline (Elavil)
        Imipramine (Tofranil)
        Doxepin (Sinequan)
        Trimipramine (Surmontil)
    Secondary amines
        Amoxapine (Asendin)
        Nortriptyline (Pamelor)
        Desipramine (Norpramin)
        Protriptyline (Vivactil)
    Tetracyclic
        Maprotiline (Ludiomil)
    Triazolopyridine
        Trazodone (Desyrel)

Monoamine Oxidase Inhibitors

Hydrazine
    Phenelzine (Nardil)
    Isocarboxazid (Marplan)
Nonhydrazine
    Tranylcypromine (Parnate)

Other Drugs

Carbamazepine (Tegretol)
Clonazepam (Klonopin, formerly Clonopin)
Clonidine (Catapres)
Meperidine (Demerol)
Methylphenidate (Ritalin)
Propranolol (Inderal)

Neuroleptics

Phenothiazines
  Aliphatics
    Chlorpromazine (Thorazine)
    Promazine (Sparine)
    Triflupromazine (Vesprin)
  Piperidine
    Thioridazine (Mellaril)
    Piperacetazine (Quide)
    Mesoridazine (Serentil)
  Piperazine
    Acetophenazine (Tindel)
    Perphenazine (Trilafon)
    Prochlorperazine (Compazine)
    Fluphenazine (Prolixin)
    Trifluoperazine (Stelazine)
Nonphenothiazines
  Thioxanthene
    Chlorprothixene (Taractan)
    Thiothixene (Navane)
  Butyrophenone
    Haloperidol (Haldol)
  Dihydroindolone
    Molindone (Moban)
  Dibenzoxazepine
    Loxapine (Loxitane)

6

Psychoanalysis and Multiple Personality Disorder

Cornelia B. Wilbur, M.D.

6

Psychoanalysis and Multiple Personality Disorder

When Berman (1981) reviewed the psychoanalytic literature for discussions of multiple personality, he found the subject sparsely represented in modern literature. He commented specifically on the limited attention given in recent years to theoretical aspects, finding this surprising and lamentable in light of renewed interest in the subject.

Ellenberger (1970) and Berman (1981) provide reviews of the history of multiple personality and "splitting" in 19th and 20th century psychoanalysis. Some important developments include the following:

1. Early theoretical and clinical work by Janet (1889) and Prince (1906) proposed mechanisms for splitting and drew a relationship between dissociation and childhood trauma.
2. Interest in the subject by Freud and Breuer later diminished on Freud's part as he came into increasing ideological conflict with Janet and moved farther from Breuer—this event directed Freud's followers away from interest in the subject.
3. Later development of the ego concept by Freud (Hartmann 1956) and Anna Freud (1936) included the existence of a relationship between ego defenses and certain illnesses.

4. Other, more recent approaches that Berman (1981) felt would open the way to theoretical understanding of multiple personality include Fairbairn's (1952) object relations theory, Kernberg's (1975) discussions of borderline conditions and narcissism, and Kohut's (1971) proposal of "vertical splitting."

During the past decade, another development has enhanced understanding of multiple personality disorder (MPD) by orders of magnitude. Increased recognition of MPD brought documentation of an overwhelming etiological association with childhood trauma, especially severe child abuse (Braun 1985; Coons 1985; Goodwin 1985; Kluft 1984; Putnam 1983). In discussing the psychoanalysis of MPD, Marmer (1980) pointed out that childhood trauma is central and causal.

Lampl-de Groot (1981) stated that many patients with MPD are analyzable if the analyst prudently screens potential patients, has the necessary patience to carry out a long and arduous therapeutic task, and has empathic capacity to understand the experiential world of the infant.

Therapeutic Considerations

Ten methods of ego defense that are described in the theoretical writings of psychoanalysis can be found in MPD. These are regression, repression, reaction formation, isolation, undoing, projection, introjection, turning against self, reversal, and sublimation.

Regression. Analysts who have worked with MPD patients are familiar with the appearance of "younger members" of the constellation of alternate personalities. These personalities are regressed individuals within the complex of the patient.

Repression. Intense affects that are repressed display themselves as alternate personalities. For example, in the presence of intense rage an alternate personality appears who expresses and deals with rage. This may be termed the "angry" personality.

Reaction Formation. Various reaction formations can be

found in MPD, as when a personality may express concern or thoughtfulness for individuals who were abusive to the patient.

Isolation.   Isolating affects from the daily life of the individual who is trying to function in society becomes the duty of personalities who deal with specific affects and their conflict.

Undoing.   A personality can undo (reverse) a painful affective response as a method of dealing with painful material.

Projection.   Multiple personality disorder patients find problems that are actually theirs vividly displayed in other people and project their feelings onto those people and situations.

Introjection.   Multiple personality disorder patients may also introject individuals or situations in an effort to deal with them. The introjects are often represented in and by personalities.

Turning Against Self.   Attempts at suicide in many MPD patients occur because the patient turns against himself or herself and turns intense affects, especially rage at past abuse, against other thought processes. Some attempts at suicide are really homicidal attempts by an angry personality against the original personality or another personality in the complex.

Reversal of Roles.   A frequent finding in MPD is the child personality being "wrong" and the abusive parent or individual being "right." Thus the patients tend to blame themselves and express intense guilt for being "bad."

Sublimation.   The usual MPD patient is an able and intelligent human being, and sublimation is not infrequent.

The most common defense in MPD is dissociation. A characteristic of many MPD patients is an ability to dissociate, manifested also as high hypnotizability. When intense anger or hatred is precipitated by a particularly cruel act, an alternate personality is formed who may then preserve all of the subsequent stimulations of violent anger and hatred. A very angry, and sometimes violent alternate may appear during analysis and try to fight with the therapist. Multiple personality disorder patients also may show phobic symptoms and avoid certain kinds of activities that they cannot tolerate. The phobia may be transferred into an alternate personality.

Multiple personality disorder patients usually enter analysis with great fear. Their most important piece of self-knowledge is that they are "different," and this difference has often led them to be uncommunicative and secretive. Establishing rapport with such patients can be difficult. A practical approach may be for the analyst to explain MPD and its effects.

Patients can be told to relate all of their thoughts, dreams, and memories as best they can, whoever they are at the time of their contact with the analyst. They can be assured that the analyst will help them to sort out intense feelings, anxieties, and fears, and to "relive" traumatic episodes so that they can be brought to the conscious mind.

The patients should be encouraged to ask any and all questions they may have about their condition. They should be brought to understand transference reactions—that at times they may react to others and to the analyst as if these individuals were those who abused them in infancy and childhood. When the patients ask about length of treatment, the analyst can only say that it will take extensive amounts of time from both patient and analyst and will probably continue over years rather than months.

The analyst must remember that any condition that precipitates intense anxiety in the patient may produce a switch to an alternate personality. In the analysis of an MPD patient the analyst may encounter alternate personalities who deal with unacceptable hatred of the abusive individual or individuals, personalities who deal with hypocrisy and dishonesty in other persons that may be intolerable to the patient, and still other personalities who deal with envy and jealousy in themselves and in others.

Different patients present conflictual material in different order. A 45-year-old woman who had suffered from MPD all her life presented first as a timid, self-conscious individual who had very little to say about herself. Shortly after she entered treatment there arrived in the office a group of "little ones" who cried profusely. An effort was made to find someone in the personality system who could inform the therapist about who was actually present in the system at the time. This is often necessary and may at times be accomplished simply by asking to speak to someone in the complex who knows about everything or who knows about the particular personality or personalities presenting. When this was done the analyst discovered a large group present, all of whom were less than nine years of age and had suffered severe trauma from a grandmother, a great-aunt, and an uncle. The traumas were all abuses of a sexual nature involving intense pain. The great-aunt was a lesbian who had a number of lesbian friends who were voyeurs. They came to watch the sexual abuses of the child over a number of days, engendering fear, pain, rage, and shame and humiliation. During the conversion of these relivings into memories the therapist was told on a number of occasions that the shame would never dissipate.

An understanding on the part of the child personality in this 45-year-old woman had to be established that the shame was not hers, that she had been abused because she was helpless, and that the great-aunt and her voyeuristic friends should suffer shame for abuse and humiliation of a helpless child. The patient also suffered feelings of guilt that somehow this had happened to her because she was "bad," as she was told by the abusive great-aunt. In addition, she feared not being believed. Fear that she would never be believed had been introduced and intensified by disbelief expressed by her mother and grandmother when she tried to tell them of the abuse. Goodwin (1985) has described the credibility problems of child abuse victims and MPD patients. The analyst's task is to elicit the patient's description, encouraging detail without seeming to be voyeuristic.

Feelings of hatred and anger may be transformed into bodily symptoms in which the patient possesses a capacity for conversion. Marmer (1980) noted that MPD must be carefully differentiated from hysteria and borderline personality disorder, with which it shares some aspects but is essentially different. Dissociation may be a seminal difference. Episodes of acute diarrhea or disturbances of the large bowel are common somatic conversions of hatred by MPD patients. Other somatic symptoms may be the result of conflicts over severe aggressive impulses.

A universal and very difficult problem in analysis of MPD patients is the presence of suicidal or homicidal personalities who may wish to do away with the original personality as the only way to deal with the intensity of hostile affects generated by abuse. Dealing with homicidal personalities, or suicidal and severely depressed personalities, necessitates dealing with the hostile affects and conflicts within the patient. Handling hostile affects within these personalities may lead to intense transference reactions on the part of the hostile personality toward the psychoanalyst. As a consequence, the therapist may be attacked verbally or even physically. Hostile alternates may criticize, condemn, annoy, yell at, and otherwise express extreme hostility toward the analyst. The attacks must be recognized as assaults in the service of transference, and the transference reactions must be analyzed in every instance. Necessarily, the abuse that created the particular transferential hostility must be sought in the analytical situation.

The analyst should not be tempted to get rid of hostile alternates by short-cutting techniques. This is not useful in terms of the succeeding life of the patient. To "get rid of" alternate personalities means to rerepress the problems that remain unsolved. Successful rerepression cannot be ensured. Consequently, the material that the hostile personalities are attempting to cope with must be analyzed.

In the presence of intense hostility and hostile transference reactions, the psychoanalyst must steadfastly remember that transference reactions are to be analyzed. Countertransference only presents the patient with a situation that he has faced many times before and usually expects to face with everyone, including the psychoanalyst. No improvement can be expected if the analyst lapses into anger with an angry personality.

Patients in psychoanalysis often become extremely dependent. Multiple personality disorder patients often become very dependent because their dependency and nurturing needs were not resolved. They are left with young alternates who express a great need for the nurturing they missed as abused infants and children. This need for nurturing and for resolution of the effects of abuse must be analyzed. Dependency must be allowed to the extent that it can be analyzed, and this gives the very young alters opportunity to mature and achieve true independence.

Analyzing dependency leads to the younger alternates' understanding their problems and need for dependency. Both the analyst and the patient come to realize that dependency can become a trap rather than a therapeutic support if the patient remains in a dependent situation, requiring the presence of the therapist in order to function. Prolonged dependency creates stress in the life of a MPD patient. It must become clear to the patient that dependency needs have to be resolved.

CONCLUSION

Psychoanalysis of the correctly diagnosed MPD patient should begin with recognition that 95 percent of such patients suffered severe abuse as children. The etiological relationship is very strong. A great many MPD patients also have high hypnotizability, a manifestation of an apparently inborn capacity to dissociate. Dissociation is the principal defense of the MPD patient against unbearable abuse, but the analyst also is likely to encounter any or all of the methods of ego defense described in the theoretical writings of psychoanalysis.

REFERENCES

Berman E: Multiple personality: psychoanalytic aspects. Int J Psychoanal 62:283–300, 1981

Braun BG: The transgenerational incidence of dissociation and multiple personality disorder: a preliminary report in Childhood Antecedents of Multiple Personality. Edited by Kluft RP. Washington, DC, American Psychiatric Press, 1985

Coons PM: Children of parents with multiple personality disorder, in Childhood Antecedents of Multiple Personality. Edited by Kluft RP. Washington, DC, American Psychiatric Press, 1985

Ellenberger HF: The Discovery of the Unconscious. New York, Basic Books, 1970

Fairbairn WRD: An Object Relations Theory of the Personality. New York, Basic Books, 1952

Freud A: The Ego and the Mechanisms of Defense. New York, International Universities Press, 1966

Goodwin J: Credibility problems in multiple personality disorder patients and abused children, in Childhood Antecedents of Multiple Personality. Edited by Kluft RP. Washington, DC, American Psychiatric Press, 1985

Hartmann H: The development of the ego concept in Freud's work. Int J Psychoanal 37:425–438, 1956

Janet P: L'Automatisme Psychologique. Paris, Bailliere, 1889

Kernberg O: Borderline Conditions and Pathological Narcissism. New York, Aronson, 1975

Kluft RP: Multiple personality in childhood, in Symposium on Multiple Personality. Edited by Braun BG. Psychiatr Clin North Am 7:121–134, 1984

Kohut H: Analysis of the Self. New York, International Universities Press, 1971

Lampl-de Groot J: Notes on multiple personality. Psychoanal Q 50:614–624, 1981

Marmer SS: Psychoanalysis of multiple personality. Int J Psychoanal 61:439–459, 1980

Prince M: Dissociation of a Personality. New York, Longman, 1906

Putnam FW, Post RM, Guroff JJ, et al: 100 cases of multiple personality disorder [New Research Abstract No. 77]. Presented at the annual meeting of the American Psychiatric Association, New York, 1983

7

Group Therapy in Treatment of Multiple Personality Disorder

David Caul, M.D.
Roberta G. Sachs, Ph.D.
Bennett G. Braun, M.D.

7

Group Therapy in Treatment of Multiple Personality Disorder

Human beings are born into a social, family environment and develop and mature in expanded hierarchies of social environments. They may suffer physical, emotional, or cognitive disabilities interwoven finely with social interaction. It is within the context of social functionability that the relief or "cure" of a disability is judged.

Humans live in groups and presumably have lived in groups for thousands of years. Our social nature was noted by Aristotle (1965 translation) when this early organizer of thought about humans and their world named man a "political animal." Among apt observations by other thinkers over the millennia is Spinoza's comment that men are scarcely able to lead a solitary life, so that to many the definition that man is a social animal must be very apparent.

The idea that humans can come together or be brought together in groups for therapeutic purposes probably has ancient roots in religious ritual and catharsis theater among other modalities that enhance a sense of belongingness. The notion of coming together in groups for specifically psychotherapeutic purposes is as old as humans' referring to their thinking about their own minds as the science of psychology.

Mesmer (Braun 1980b; Rosenbaum 1963) established formal hypnosis therapy groups in early 18th century Vienna. As equivocal a figure in science then as he is now, he was banished from the city for practicing magic. Social work pioneer Jane Addams set up community-based, reality-oriented psychotherapeutic groups in 1889 soon after opening Hull House in Chicago, thereby giving modern group psychotherapy one of its first models (Shaffer and Galinsky 1974).

In 1905 Boston internist Joseph Pratt began establishing groups for the purpose of bringing poor, socially outcast tuberculosis patients together to find a "common bond in a common disease" (Spetnitz 1961). Dr. Pratt's observations made him increasingly aware of the psychological aspects of group interaction, and today he is often called the first practitioner of modern group therapy.

Moreno (1934) initiated psychodrama in Vienna in 1910 and his "theatre of spontaneity" in 1921 as applications of his social theory of interaction. In 1932 he coined the term "group psychotherapy" (Shaffer and Galinsky 1974).

Psychoanalysts Burrows, Wender, and Schilder (Shaffer and Galinsky 1974) practiced and wrote about group psychotherapy in the 1930s.

World War II was a major impetus to development of group psychotherapy in the United States because psychotherapists in the military services had more patients than they could handle in individual therapy. Once forced into group therapy, now many therapists found the experience positive for their patients and for themselves. American and British psychiatrists began to show interest in augmenting individual therapy with group therapy. Experience with groups began to grow into theoretical constructions, such as when Foulkes and Bion (Foulkes 1965) pointed out "group process" as the significant curative factor in treatment.

Proliferation of group psychotherapy potentiated the assembling of data regarding its benefits for patients: acquisition of new knowledge, increased number of interpersonal skills and ability to apply them, identification with others who share the same disabilities, learning not to be ashamed of thoughts and emotions, giving up inappropriate defenses, learning to accept criticism without pathological interpersonal defense, learning to observe others without pathological interpersonal judgments, learning to respect the feelings of others, sharing perspectives and assisting others to resolve their difficulties, learning to feel safe in a group environment, and learning how to restructure the original family constellation in order to work on issues and abreact.

GROUP PSYCHOTHERAPY AND MULTIPLE PERSONALITY DISORDER: GENERAL CONSIDERATIONS

Expanded interest in group psychotherapy led to interest in widening the categories of patients eligible for group process. A prime criterion for establishing a group is still Dr. Pratt's "common bond."

Within the past 10 years, victims of incest and child abuse and their abusers have increasingly been viewed as patients who could benefit from group therapy. Incest and child abuse groups drew more interest as data accumulated to document the previously unacknowledged high incidence of such abuse in American society (National Committee for the Prevention of Child Abuse 1985). Goodwin (1985) pointed out the desperate need of incest and child abuse victims to be believed, to be safe, and to find others who suffered similar experiences.

Like incest and child abuse victims, MPD patients share a "common bond" of being isolated in society, not being understood or believed, and feeling worthless or deserving of the abuse they were accustomed to receiving. Experience is indeed showing that although individual therapy is the mode of choice, carefully selected and screened MPD patients can realize benefits in groups that enhance and facilitate the therapeutic process. Multiple personality patients rarely have had the opportunity or ability to understand the concepts of self and self in the world. Group therapy presents an opportunity for the MPD patient to participate in a sense of togetherness with other humans in a social context. The group presents a potential to learn interaction, acceptance, tolerance, patience, compassion, sharing. Caul (1984) believes the therapist is obliged to open these opportunities for the MPD patient whenever possible.

Group Setting and Composition

Scientific literature on group therapy of MPD patients is not extensive. Multiple personality disorder was considered a rare condition until *DSM–III* legitimatized its diagnosis; thus few therapists had access to enough patients to even consider starting a group. Those therapists who were familiar with MPD were not necessarily advocates of group therapy; the characteristic isolation, secretive behavior, dissociation, and "switching" episodes of MPD patients made them seem to some therapists less than desirable persons to place in a group.

The first inpatient MPD group was started by Caul in 1976. Braun and Sachs started the first outpatient group in 1978, and Coons and Bradley started the second in 1980 (Coons and Bradley 1985). Review of their experiences and that of clinicians who followed provides some insights into groups organized in inpatient or outpatient settings with MPD patients constituting all or part of the group members.

Homogeneous Groups

Sachs and Braun (1985) noted that when they started their MPD group they made an assumption that proved to be erroneous regardless of whether an MPD group was homogeneous, heterogeneous, inpatient, or outpatient. They assumed that the diagnosis of MPD alone was an indication for a patient's selection. However, MPD is a diagnosis within which exists a continuum from high-level-functioning patients who are well along in therapy to severely polyfragmented patients who are barely functional. Also in conjunction with MPD other *DSM–III* diagnoses are commonly found (Putnam 1984). Sachs and Braun, and Coons and Bradley eventually concluded that high-level-functioning MPD patients who have considerable experience in individual psychotherapy are the best candidates for group process. High-level-functioning and low-level-functioning MPD patients placed in the same ongoing outpatient group will not have many of their therapeutic needs met.

The diagnostic criteria of *DSM–III* provide an initial screen to ensure MPD selection. Patients also should be screened for indications of borderline personality disorder, not an easy task given that as many as 70 percent of MPD patients may also meet *DSM–III* diagnostic criteria for borderline personality (Horevitz and Braun 1984). Multiple personality/borderline patients without sufficient treatment can be so disruptive that they are now excluded from the Braun and Sachs group, and Coons and Bradley warn strongly of their potential disruptiveness in groups.

Even patients who have been carefully screened for diagnosis and level of functioning should not be placed in group psychotherapy unless they are concomitantly in individual therapy (Coons and Bradley 1985; Sachs and Braun 1985). Group process is a supplement to individual therapy for MPD patients, not a modality that could or should be used alone.

The first two years of the seven-year experience reported by Sachs and Braun (1985) with their group of nine outpatients that they thought was homogeneous was a virtual exposition of Murphy's Law. Coons has said that reports of Sachs and Braun's experience helped him avoid or mitigate some problems in forming his and Bradley's group. A therapist may anticipate that the MPD patient's life history and narcissistic investment in multiplicity will appear in group therapy as sibling rivalry, somatization, dissociation, switching, greater to lesser degrees of abreaction, and competition for dominance. Patients can and do use their multiplicity "skills" to compete for honors as the "best" multiple personality patient in the group. Caul (1984) said that in his experience with MPD groups, achieving group cohesiveness and direction was a difficult, labor-intensive, and frustrating undertaking. Some MPD patients can make significant therapeutic progress in groups, however, only if both the patients and therapist(s) are willing to invest the requisite time and effort.

A group should not be initiated without the therapist's firmly stating and enforcing rules outlining behavior boundaries between group members and therapists, time structure of group meetings, safety within the group, and specific limits on individual behaviors. Stressed again and again must be the issues of honesty and confidentiality, both of which are of great concern to patients whose lives have been spent in secrecy and fear.

Pseudointimacy between patients and therapists can develop early on and slow group progress unless interpreted and worked through. The problem of individual therapy occurring during group time is another compelling phenomenon that can slow the group's progress. A proper balance of limits, boundaries, intimacy (see Chapter 1 of this book), and individual/group therapy ratio must be found.

Videotaping of group sessions (Caul 1984) is a valuable procedure for documenting switching episodes. Patients are seldom if ever offended by video feedback after switching, and the group process can be enhanced. Video also serves as a tool for the therapist to review individual and group process; it maintains the subtle nuances that notes lose, but it does take more time to review.

Sachs and Braun (1985) and Caul (1984) have successfully used hypnosis in the homogeneous group setting to control impulses, switches, and somatization.

The need for cotherapists is strongly agreed upon by Sachs and Braun (1985), Coons and Bradley (1985), Scobey et al. (1985), and Mason and Brownback (1985). Points of agreement on cotherapy include the following:

- Hostile transference to one therapist can be interrupted by the other.
- One therapist can observe while the other works.
- One therapist can serve the other as an "island of sanity."
- A female cotherapist can deflect and direct to its appropriate target the anger that a patient may display toward a male therapist who he or she perceives as a father figure.
- Cotherapists can and should plan group strategies, process jointly after group sessions, assist one another in record keeping, and protect one another against burnout.
- Cotherapists should help patients learn new coping skills by working out in group sessions their disagreements on therapy, thus serving as role models for patients who have no such skills.

Cotherapists must respect and trust one another. Patients can detect any dislike or competitiveness between therapists and quickly form "us versus them" subgroups. The problem of "us versus them" may be enhanced when one or two patients are in individual therapy with a physician other than one of the cotherapists. Regular consultations with the outside therapist are a must to maintain the patient's progress and mitigate group tensions.

Sachs and Braun (1985) and Coons and Bradley (1985) use and recommend the here-and-now group process described by Yalom (1975). They find this ahistorical approach most useful in the difficult task of building group cohesion, establishing rapport, diminishing isolation of patients, and eliminating the patient's lifelong fear of his or her "freakishness."

Heterogeneous Groups

Caul (1984) reported on groups of inpatients that included MPD patients as members and commented that they can be highly disruptive in a heterogeneous setting. Inpatient groups are sometimes heterogeneous simply because there are not enough MPD patients in an institution to make up a homogeneous group. In Caul's study, the non-MPD patients considered the MPD patients to be self-centered and malingering; the MPD patients saw the non-MPD patients as uncaring and rejecting.

Mason and Brownback (1985) reported the discovery of two previously undiagnosed MPD patients in a heterogeneous group and discussed their reasons for leaving the patients in the group, which were as follows:

- They anticipated a potentially negative impact on the MPD patient if he or she was dismissed from the group and the feeling of cohesion it affords.
- Other group members wanted the newly discovered MPD patient to stay.
- They anticipated positive therapeutic effects of the MPD patient's sharing of his or her diagnosis with the group.
- Switching by an MPD patient allowed another group member to role-play a child in need of the nurturing not received in childhood.
- Revelation of sexual abuse by an MPD patient opened the way to another patient's disclosure of sexual abuse as a child.
- Even though extra therapist time was required, other patients' responses to MPD were dealt with in a structured and therapeutically useful group process.

Braun also discovered two MPD patients in a heterogeneous group. He did not find their inclusion in the group to be a problem; however, these two MPD patients were high functioning. Bowers et al. (1971) found group therapy useful for their MPD patient.

Caul's experience with general groups in a hospital setting indicated that MPD patients and others were often mutually intolerant in group therapy, although some were able to establish positive relationships outside of the group. He believed that an MPD patient who is struggling with therapy may find a general group a difficult or negative experience but that an integrated or co-conscious patient can benefit. Braun and Sachs, working in the Dissociative Disorders Program at Rush-Presbyterian-St. Luke's Medical Center in Chicago, have experienced a similar phenomenon but find that MPD patients can participate in task-oriented groups.

One-upmanship practiced by MPD patients was a constant sore spot with non-MPD patients, who found their stories constantly "topped" by the MPD patients' life stories. "Topping" led to isolation of the MPD patients by the non-MPD patients.

Trust and confidentiality are a severe problem for MPD patients in heterogeneous groups. The typically secretive, nontrusting MPD patient is likely to project, distort, misinterpret, or take literally the words and actions of other group members.

Goodwin (1985) and Summit (1982) recommend the value of special-purpose child abuse and incest groups. For some carefully selected MPD patients, the experience helps to further reduce isolation and feelings of negative self-worth.

Internal Group Therapy

The technique of internal group therapy is described by Caul (1984) as an alternative and/or supportive modality for the patient whose multiplicity is well defined, who is well along in individual psychotherapy, and who is capable of coordinating a group therapy session with a selected group of his or her own personalities. The therapist's role is that of silent observer. He or she may also initiate the session with hypnosis, if the patient is unable to easily reach the personalities and facilitate smooth switching for the internal group session. Caul has found that therapeutic progress may increase shortly after an internal group therapy session that was videotaped was reviewed later by the patient and therapist. This helps promote co-consciousness.

Internal group therapy should be undertaken only if the therapist is sure that the patient fully understands the process. According to Caul, the therapist should do four things:

1. Conduct an interview with the patient to explain the process and judge the patient's willingness and understanding.

2. Explain that the patient will control the session, determining which personality will be in charge and which others will attend, what topics will be discussed, how long the session will last, and how it will be brought to a close.
3. Explain that the therapist will have no role other than silent observation but will be available for emergencies.
4. Explain that the session will be videotaped for later viewing with the therapist.

GENERAL CONSIDERATIONS FOR THERAPISTS

No issue has more meaning to the MPD patient in group psychotherapy than trust. The patient whose primary psychological defense is dissociation and whose most characteristic appearance before the world is one of secrecy, narcissism, and isolation cannot reap the benefits of group cohesion and process if he or she does not learn trust. Even the first appearance of trust may be illusory. Coons and Bradley (1985) saw an initial euphoria among members of a newly "cohered" MPD group turn to mistrust soon after. Solid trust and cohesion as opposed to pseudointimacy may be a matter of additional months, a year, or more. The building of trust lies in the approach and relationship of the therapists, in patient selection and screening, and in open, honest working together over time.

The importance of co-therapists is strongly agreed on among those with the longest group experience (Coons and Bradley 1985; Sachs and Braun 1985; Scobey et al. 1985). Sachs and Braun emphasize that the therapists should have a good relationship, probably one that originated before the group was initiated. They should be truly co-therapists and not therapist and assistant, or patients will be quick to detect and exploit via splitting the boss/assistant relationship; they should be of opposite sexes, although Scobey et al. (1985) disagree on that point; they should meet before every session to prepare an agenda and after every session to process; and they should be alert for burnout symptoms in one another and aware of the powerful effects of transference and countertransference.

As general considerations for group psychotherapy for MPD patients, we suggest the following:
1. Co-therapists should jointly screen group MPD candidates according to *DSM–III* criteria and should be aware of the

possibility of borderline personality disorder as an over-lapping diagnosis.

2. Limit group size to six at first. Eight may work with the proper patients and experienced leaders.
3. Misdiagnosed MPD patients may be kept in a heterogeneous group to work through significant issues, but if they are unrelentingly disruptive they must be asked to leave the group.
4. Misdiagnosed non-MPD patients in an MPD group may benefit from the group if they have a related dissociative disorder, but if they are malingering they will be disruptive.
5. Group members should thoroughly understand the concepts of group psychotherapy, especially the importance of honesty and confidentiality.
6. Group members must all be in individual therapy.
7. Group members should work with therapists to set therapeutic goals.
8. Here-and-now group process as described by Yalom (1975) is the mode of choice: Using a two-tiered approach, the group members must 1) focus their attention on their feelings toward group members and the therapist rather than on historical events, and 2) study its interpersonal transactions in a self-reflective process.
9. Role playing and behavior rehearsal may be used to prepare patients for events outside the group.
10. Therapists should not facilitate abreactions in group.
11. Interventions such as hypnosis may be used, but only if the therapists are comfortable in doing so. Hypnotic interventions that have been described by Braun (1980a, 1984a) and Kluft (1982) may be adopted for group use.

CONCLUSION

Group psychotherapy is a useful adjunct to individual psychotherapy of patients with MPD when applied with carefully diagnosed and screened patients within recognized limitations and especially within well-defined rules, boundaries, and timelines.

REFERENCES

Aristotle: Politics and Poetics. Translated by Jowett, Twining. New York, Viking Press, 1965

Bowers MK, Brecher-Marer S, Newton BW, et al: Theory of multiple personality. Int J Clin Exp Hypn 19:57–65, 1971

Braun BG: Hypnosis for multiple personalities, in Clinical Hypnosis in Medicine. Edited by Wain HF. Chicago, Year Book Publishers, 1980a

Braun BG: Hypnosis in groups and group hypnotherapy, in Handbook of Hypnosis and Psychosomatic Medicine. Edited by Burrows G, Dennerstein L. Amsterdam, Elsevier/North Holland Biomedical Press, 1980b

Braun BG: Uses of hypnosis with multiple personality. Psychiatric Annals 14:34–40, 1984a

Caul D: Group and videotape techniques for multiple personality. Psychiatric Annals 14:43–50, 1984

Coons PM: Children of parents with multiple personality disorder, in Childhood Antecedents of Multiple Personality. Edited by Kluft RP. Washington, DC, American Psychiatric Press, 1985

Coons PM, Bradley K: Group psychotherapy with multiple personality patients. J Nerv Ment Dis 173:515–521, 1985

Foulkes SH: Therapeutic Group Analysis. New York, International Universities Press, 1965

Goodwin J: Credibility problems in multiple personality disorder patients and abused children, in Childhood Antecedents of Multiple Personality. Edited by Kluft RP. Washington, DC, American Psychiatric Press, 1985

Horevitz RP, Braun BG: Are multiple personalities borderline? in Symposium on Multiple Personality. Edited by Braun BG. Psychiatr Clin North Am 7:69–87, 1984

Kluft RP: Multiple personality in childhood, in Symposium on Multiple Personality. Edited by Braun BG. Psychiatr Clin North Am 7:121–134, 1984

Kluft RP: Varieties of hypnotherapeutic interventions in the treatment of multiple personality. Am J Clin Hypn 24:230–240, 1982

Mason LA, Brownback TS: The emergence of two multiple personalities in a group: a description and assessment, in Dissociative Disorders 1985: Proceedings of the Second International Conference on Multiple Personality/Dissociated States. Edited by Braun BG. Chicago, Rush University, 1985

Moreno JL: Who Shall Survive? Washington, DC, Nervous and Mental Disease Publishing Company, 1934

National Committee for the Prevention of Child Abuse: The size of the child abuse problem (NCPCA Working Paper No. 8). Chicago, NCPCA Publishing Department, 1985

Putnam FW, Lowenstein RJ, Silberman EJ, et al: Multiple personality disorder in a hospital setting. J Clin Psychiatry 45:172–175, 1984

Rosenbaum M, Berger M (Eds.): Group Psychotherapy and Group Function. New York, Basic Books, 1963

Sachs RG, Braun BG: The evolution of an outpatient multiple personality disorder group: A seven-year study, in Dissociation Disorders 1985: Proceedings of the Second International Conference on Multiple Personality/Dissociative States. Edited by Braun BG. Chicago, Rush University, 1985

Scobey J, Kelley P, Parr B: The use of group co-therapy for multiple personality disorder, in Dissociative Disorders 1985: Proceedings of the Second International Conference on Multiple Personality/Dissociative States. Edited by Braun BG. Chicago, Rush University, 1985

Shaffer J, Galinsky MD: Models of Group Therapy and Sensitivity Training. Englewood Cliffs, NJ, Prentice-Hall, 1974

Spetnitz H: The Couch and the Circle. New York, Alfred Knopf, 1961

Spinoza B: Ethics and On the Correction of the Understanding. Translated by Boyle. New York, Dutton Everyman's Library, 1977

Stern CR: The etiology of multiple personalities, in Symposium on Multiple Personality. Edited by Braun BG. Psychiatr Clin North Am 7:149–159, 1984

Summit R: The reluctant discovery of incest, in Women's Sexual Experiences. Edited by Kilpatrick M. New York, Plenum, 1982

Yalom ID: The Theory and Practice of Psychotherapy (Second Edition). New York, Basic Books, 1975

8

The Adjunctive Role of Social Support Systems in the Treatment of Multiple Personality Disorder

Roberta G. Sachs, Ph.D.

8

The Adjunctive Role of
Social Support Systems
in the Treatment of
Multiple Personality Disorder

The past 20 years have witnessed a growing recognition of the role that social support systems play in the successful treatment of a wide variety of psychiatric disorders. For example, the existence of positive social support systems has been found to be an important factor in the rehabilitation of alcoholics (Finney and Moos 1981), chronic schizophrenics (Brown et al. 1972), and others suffering from postpartum depression (Cutrona 1984). It seems logical then to presume that the role of social support systems may also have a beneficial effect in the treatment of multiple personality disorder (MPD).

A BRIEF DESCRIPTION OF
MULTIPLE PERSONALITY DISORDER

Multiple personality disorder is one of four dissociative disorders listed in the current *Diagnostic and Statistical Manual of Mental Disorders* (*Third Edition*) (*DSM–III*; American Psychiatric Association 1980). The essential feature of such disorders is a sudden and temporary alteration in the normally integrative functions of consciousness, identity, and/or motor behavior. Three criteria distinguish MPD from other dissociative disorders; 1) the existence of two or more distinct personality states, each of which is dominant at a particular time; 2) the personality state that is dominant has executive control over the individual's behavior; and 3) each personality state is complex and integrated with its own unique behavior patterns and social relationships. Braun (1985) cogently argued that each of these three criteria should be observed consistently over time before the diagnosis of MPD can be formally made.

The 3-P Model of Multiple Personality Disorder

In order to illustrate how various support systems can be adjunctively utilized in the treatment of MPD, a clinical model (Braun and Sachs 1985) is described here. (For a diagram of the model, see Chapter 1). The model is called the 3-P model of MPD because it focuses on the predisposing, precipitating, and perpetuating factors that are associated with the development of this syndrome. Each type of factor in the model will be considered separately.

Predisposing Factors. Two predisposing factors for the development of MPD have been identified: 1) an inborn dissociative capacity and 2) a psychosocial environment characterized by consistent but unpredictable physical and psychological trauma. It is necessary for both of these factors to be present for the individual to develop MPD. Neither alone is sufficient. Individuals with dissociative ability who are not exposed to bizarre and unpredictable abuse typically become normal highly hypnotizable individuals. In contrast children with little or no dissociative capacity who are exposed to such abuse are likely to manifest some type of psychiatric disorder other than MPD.

Most often it is the family environment that is the source of the inconsistent and overwhelming trauma. While other sources of trauma can sometimes also be identified, in the majority of patients studied so far, the source of the trauma is typically found in the family environment. One salient feature of the abuse that occurs in the family environment of an individual who later develops MPD is that it is consistent but unpredictable. For example, a child may be severely beaten or affectionately hugged on different occasions for the same behavior. This unpredictable abuse becomes so traumatic that the individual with dissociative capacity surrounds all memories associated with the trauma with an amnestic barrier. Because different memory systems do not have access to all the knowledge stored in each system, the ego is ready to be partitioned into independent information processing systems.

Precipitating Factors. The occurrence of a single highly traumatic event that triggers a chaining between a number of dissociated memories is the precipitating factor in the development of MPD. These separate dissociated memories become integrated by a common theme. For example, a child who has been forced to endure repeated and sadistic physical abuse one day becomes enraged and begins to physically retaliate. The child's collective memories of parental rape become the impetus for initiating a new adaptive response. This response appears uncharacteristic of the child's behavior from past observation. In addition, the personality state that typically has executive control of the body (the host personality) is usually unaware of this new behavior and denies any knowledge of it. However, these previously dissociated memories have now become united by a potential solution to a common problem and begin to take on a life history of their own. Over time, this develops into a personality fragment with a particular adaptive function that is not part of the behavioral repertoire of the host personality.

Up to this point, the consciousness of this newly created personality fragment has only past memories for events that are connected by this one unifying theme. In addition, the memory for the new adaptive response is added to these earlier memories. However, although this fragment has an unconscious adaptive function, it is not yet a separate fully developed personality state.

Perpetuating Factors. In order for a full personality state to coalesce, the united memories of the fragment begin to form a self-consciousness that begins to actively respond to situations in the host personality's everyday life space. The host personality is usually unaware of the fact that it no longer has executive control of the body all of the time. Factors that repeatedly stimulate this personality fragment to take executive control of the body have been identified as perpetuating phenomena in the development of MPD. These factors promote further

switching and splitting and facilitate the development of a separate life history. When a fragment develops its own life history
along with a wide range of its own cognitions and emotions, a
new personality state has been created. The perpetuating phenomena are typically related to the predisposing and precipitating factors that preceded the creation of the new personality
state. That is, the same traumatic and unpredictable environment that first stimulated the use of dissociation as a defense
maintains and promotes the development of one or more new
personality states. This observation has been acknowledged by
almost all clinicians who have treated several cases of MPD
(Braun and Sachs 1985; Fagan and McMahon 1984; Kluft 1984a,
1984b; Kluft et al. 1985; Wilbur 1984).

Implications of the 3-P Model for Social Support Interventions

Multiple personality disorder is strongly related to the patient's
preexisting social systems. However, trying to shelter the patient
from these pernicious influences does not lead to a reversal of
the symptom progression. For example, there is strong evidence
that MPD patients continue to seek environments and situations
that are similar to the ones that stimulated the development of
the syndrome (Braun 1985). This self-defeating behavior promotes further splitting and switching and perpetuates the development of MPD.

The above consideration indicates that the primary treatment
approach should focus on the patient rather than the environment. However, it is sometimes necessary to protect patients
from their insidious environments. This is where social support
systems can be a valuable adjunct in the treatment process. The
3-P model has several implications for the role of social support
systems in treating MPD.

The 3-P model identifies the family environment as the most
likely source of the trauma that promoted the development of
MPD. This observation is valid in almost all cases seen. Parents,
grandparents, and siblings are typically the source of the psychosocial and physical abuse, suggesting that some type of family or marital intervention would be beneficial. The nature of
the intervention should relate to the current age and psychosocial development of the MPD patient.

FAMILY INTERVENTIONS

When a Child Is the Identified Multiple Personality Disorder Patient

The existence of childhood MPD has now been documented by several different clinicians (Fagan and McMahon 1984; Kluft 1984b). This should not seem surprising since the 3-P model predicts that the source of the trauma that caused this syndrome to develop is typically precipitated by family interactions in the patient's early childhood. Therefore, it is important to observe, document, and understand the nature of these relationships.

Several clinicians have now reported on the role of the family and intrafamilial abuse in the development of MPD (Braun 1985; Kluft et al. 1985; Wilbur 1984). These reports have all noted that the family of origin of an MPD patient is likely to present as a "united front" (Kramer 1968), as though all were well except for the problems of the identified patient. The parents try to represent the family environment as being normal and sometimes as being ideal. Any questioning of the validity of this "pseudo-normal veneer" (Kluft el al. 1985) is interpreted as an affront and vehemently denied. However, repeated observation typically reveals that the family environment is nothing like the image that was initially projected. At this point, the parents begin to rationalize about incidents that are contrary to their earlier descriptions.

How should the therapist intervene in such a case? First, he or she must make certain that the cycle of abuse is stopped. One cannot overemphasize the importance of this objective, because any therapeutic attempt is useless unless the abuse is terminated. The therapist must address this issue directly, and parents must be confronted about the abuse. In addition, recent legal decisions (Abused and Neglected Child Reporting Act 1980) have mandated that the therapist notify the Department of Family Services if any type of child abuse is suspected. If the parents continue to deny the abuse in the face of cumulative evidence to the contrary, then steps must be immediately taken to make the family environment safe. If this cannot be done, then the child must be removed from the home to prevent the perpetuation of dissociation.

Four criteria must be met before a family intervention is

deemed viable for a childhood MPD patient. First, the abuser(s) must be identified. Second, the abuser(s) must be willing to admit to the abuse. Third, the abuser(s) must be willing to change. Finally, there must also be some means for verifying that the abuse cycle has been stopped. If any of these criteria are not met, then a family intervention will probably not be effective because the possibility of further abuse still remains.

At this point an example will prove illustrative. I once treated a family who had recently experienced a divorce. The father had received custody of the children, and the mother did not participate in any of the therapy sessions. There were five children in the family, and therapy proceeded for approximately eight months before it was discontinued for logistic reasons. After treatment was terminated, the eldest daughter called me and expressed an interest in entering individual psychotherapy. Unfortunately, a year went by before she was able to begin. During the first year of therapy, it became apparent that this patient was suffering from MPD. I learned that she and her siblings had been severely beaten by their father for revelations they had made in the context of family therapy years earlier. This had been unknown at the time and clearly illustrates what can happen if the abuse is not identified and monitored. On the surface, the father had admitted to some inappropriate disciplinary actions that the children had mentioned during the course of family therapy. He had also pledged that he would do his best to see that these did not reoccur. However, upon returning home, the children had been severely punished for their revelations, and the abuse cycle actually had escalated instead of ending.

This example underscores the necessity of monitoring the abuse cycle. The father, in this case, said one thing and did another. Clearly, the therapist must find some way to verify that the abuse has been stopped so that the effectiveness of individual treatment can be maximized. If the abuser is willing to admit to what he or she has done and is willing to change, and evidence that the abuse has stopped can be verified, then it is possible to incorporate the treatment of the child MPD patient along with the treatment of the abuser.

How can a family intervention prove useful for the childhood MPD patient? First, the home environment must be modified so that there is a consistent, predictable, and nurturing family atmosphere. This promotes the development of different adaptive responses on the part of the child. Second, limits and boundaries must be set to facilitate safety and to provide a general message of love and support for the child. Childhood MPD patients must learn that they will be loved no matter what they do. For example, if a destructive and violent personality takes executive control of a child's body, one of the parents can protectively hold the child to keep the child from hurting himself or herself or others. In this manner, child MPD patients will come to learn that they will not be allowed to hurt themselves and that no matter how much acting out takes place, they will still be loved. If these suggestions can be implemented, then a family intervention will prove to be an effective adjunct to the treatment of the childhood MPD patient.

When a Parent Is the Identified Multiple Personality Disorder Patient

When the MPD patient is married and has a family, a family intervention is beneficial for two reasons. First, it allows the therapist to explore the family environment for signs of potential stress which may be causing the patient to switch or dissociate on the home front. Second, it allows the therapist to examine the impact of the parental psychopathology on the children. Each of these issues will be discussed separately.

It is likely that the MPD patient who has a family frequently switches personalities while in the home. Since the process of switching is not random, it is useful to explore the family environment in order to identify potential sources of stress which trigger the switching process. Once this has been done, appropriate therapeutic interventions can focus on modifying these problem areas. If one of the problem areas concerns the relationship between the spouses, then marital therapy should also be considered. This possibility will be discussed later.

Since the MPD patient grew up in a family environment characterized by overwhelming and unpredictable trauma, the patient is likely to reenact some of the maladaptive responses that he or she was exposed to as a child. It has been theorized that we tend to repeat our childhoods when we ourselves become parents (Kempe and Kempe 1978). In addition, the impact of patental modeling on subsequent child development has been clearly demonstrated (Bandura 1977). Finally, a transgenerational study (Braun 1985) suggests that the genetic and environmental influence of parents can have a dramatic impact on the development of MPD. These considerations suggest that the therapist should carefully assess the children of an MPD patient in order to identify any potential signs of incipient MPD (Kluft 1984b).

It is always essential to check whether the MPD parent is abusing his or her children. If this is the case, then the abuse cycle must be stopped or actions must be taken by the therapist to remove the children from the MPD parent's sphere of influence. The therapist must directly confront the MPD parent with this issue. At this point, contracting is useful. In addition, it is necessary to structure some type of accountability with either one or the other parent or the child in order to ensure that the abuse has ceased. This can also be the beginning of a forum for helping the MPD patient begin to deal with parenting issues.

Another implication of the above considerations is that a family intervention can help the children to deal with their MPD parent. At this point, it is helpful and often necessary to validate the childrens' perception of their parent. It is true that this parent does change. The children are usually aware of this fact, but they do not understand it. For example, it is difficult for them to comprehend why they get different reactions on different occasions for the same behavior. The therapist must validate the childrens' perception of reality and help them to understand that their parent's inconsistent behavior is due to an illness and that other parents do not behave as their parent does. This has the potential for strengthening the ego of the children and makes it less likely that they will imitate the MPD parent's behavior.

The Multiple Personality Disorder Patient in Marital Therapy

If the MPD patient is married, then marital therapy can be an important adjunct to the primary treatment approach. This facilitates the survival of the marriage and promotes the ultimate integration of the MPD patient.

Marital therapy should deal with here-and-now issues. These

include educating the spouse about the nature of MPD and preparing the spouse to expect changes as the primary treatment progresses. This helps the spouse to understand the cyclical patterns of behavior that are exhibited by his or her partner. As therapy progresses, the MPD patient should be encouraged to share information about his or her problems instead of having the therapist inform the spouse. This promotes further sharing, helps to build trust, and strengthens the relationship.

Several caveats are necessary when considering marital therapy. First, if the MPD patient has married someone who reminded him or her of an abusive parent, the therapist should check to see if the patient's spouse is abusive in the marital relationship. If so, then marital therapy must immediately focus on stopping this abuse. If the abuse cannot be stopped, then steps must be taken to isolate the patient from his or her spouse, such as hospitalization without visitation rights. Remember, the primary treatment is useless if the patient is still being abused.

Another caveat to consider when doing marital therapy is that the spouse may be sabotaging the primary treatment. This can occur in several ways. First the spouse may act as a lay therapist and try to manipulate the various personalities so that his or her needs are met. In this case, the therapist must intervene and inform the spouse of the potential negative consequences of this behavior. Second, the spouse may fear the loss of favored personalities. In this case, the therapist needs to address the spouse's fear. The therapist should inform the spouse that the characteristics of favored personalities will eventually emerge after integration has been achieved. If each of the above caveats are addressed in marital therapy, then the progress of the primary treatment can be facilitated and psychological integration may be expedited.

OTHER POTENTIAL SUPPORT SYSTEMS

In this section, I will consider how the therapist can adjunctively utilize other potential support systems to facilitate the MPD patient's further progress in individual treatment. These include various parenting and incest programs, assertiveness training groups, the clergy, peer networks, substance abuse groups, leisure activity groups, vocational counselors, various tutorial groups, and 24-hour hotlines. The common feature of these systems is that they promote healthy social interaction with other people in a safe environment.

Parenting Programs

Parenting programs provide education about parenting issues. Of particular interest is the teaching of appropriate child developmental schedules. Inappropriate parental expectations are one of the main causes of child abuse (Kempe and Kempe 1978). For example, one MPD parent confessed that she had beaten her child for not being toilet trained by the age of two. The parent complained that the child had been shown how to use the toilet but failed to do so. Closer examination revealed that the child was much too young to understand toilet training skills.

Parenting programs provide information about when children can be expected to sit, crawl, speak, or be toilet trained. They also focus on appropriate disciplinary actions and the concept of punishment. For example, until age two the child may not be capable of comprehending the concept of punishment. Any type of physical discipline administered before this age can be considered a form of abuse. Age-appropriate disciplinary skills are emphasized in most parenting programs. It should not be assumed that parents already possess these skills. In many cases MPD parents do not have the knowledge necessary to develop them.

Parenting programs are useful for MPD parents because they help correct preconceived notions about developmental issues that were learned from their parents. Most MPD patients have a history of abuse from early childhood. Parenting programs teach that abuse is not normal, which is often a revelation to the typical MPD parent. Such programs are also task/skill oriented and give the MPD parent a chance to practice appropriate disciplinary actions with supervised behavioral rehearsal.

Parents Anonymous

Parents Anonymous is a nationwide child abuse program. One of the main components of this organization is parent support groups that are run by trained leaders. The leaders facilitate group discussion about issues such as the lack of impluse control and what child behaviors trigger abuse. In addition, there are also child support groups for children of abusive parents. These groups allow children to express their feelings in a safe environment. Both the parent and child support groups focus on the identification and expression of feelings surrounding affectively charged topics.

One of the most effective safeguards against further abuse involves getting both parents to attend these group meetings. This helps to build a sense of accountability into the family system. Specific contracts can be made in the presence of other parents that will foster a safe environment for the child. For example, if the parent has made a contract to stop abusing but in reality continues to abuse, the other parent will be obligated to phone the police.

One potential caveat needs to be mentioned about Parents Anonymous groups and their appropriateness for MPD patients. Remember that MPD patients were inconsistently and often sadistically abused when they were children. Some of the highly charged group material may trigger abreactions of this original trauma. Therefore, the primary therapist should contract with the MPD patient about which personality state will attend the group and what is to be done if the group affect becomes overwhelming.

Incest Groups

Incest groups are for people who have been sexually abused by a family member. The groups promote sharing the "secret of incest" in a safe environment and facilitate the ventilation of intense feelings caused by highly traumatic issues. Putnam et al. (1983) and Schultz et al. (1985) independently reported an extremely high incidence of sexual abuse for MPD patients. More than 95 percent of the patients in each of these studies had some history of sexual abuse. The sharing of this trauma with other abuse victims is usually very therapeutic. However, several considerations are necessary before a therapist should encourage an MPD patient to attend an incest group. First, the value of sharing traumatic material is beneficial only if the MPD patient is stable and functioning at a moderate to high level. Group issues often reinstate memories that trigger the switching of personalities. These personalities may respond with escalating fear and anger that may disrupt group functioning. The primary therapist must decide if the MPD patient is ready to deal with such possibilities.

Another consideration about an MPD patient's attending an incest group is which personality state will go to the meetings. The MPD patient must be far enough along in his or her primary treatment that a contract can be made about who will attend. These personalities will selectively filter information to others. It may also be helpful if the patient or the primary therapist informs the group leader about the MPD diagnosis. With this knowledge, the group leader can be better prepared to facilitate group interactions.

Assertiveness Training Groups

Assertiveness training groups can be useful adjuncts to the primary treatment of MPD if the patient has reached a high enough level of adaptive functioning. Such groups teach constructive confrontation skills with behavioral rehearsal under the supervision of a person who is capable of giving the patient positive feedback about his or her performance. Thus the MPD patient can behviorally learn how to make a point and how to protect himself or herself verbally without assaulting another person's feelings. The purpose of assertiveness training is to teach the MPD patient how to transform rage into constructive anger that will get positive results for the person who is expressing it.

The Clergy

Members of the clergy can often be useful as supportive listeners in addition to the primary therapist and other support systems. However, because most clergy members are viewed as authority figures, it is particularly important that the MPD patient share the diagnosis. The clergy member must understand that most MPD patients have a past history of being abused by authority figures. The clergy member's role is to be an empathic listener and not a psychotherapist.

Peer Networks

Informal MPD peer networks are now beginning to form on a nationwide basis ("Speaking for Ourselves," a newsletter published in Long Beach, California, is one example). The purpose of these networks is to allow MPD patients to talk to each other. This is often useful in the beginning of treatment and helps to diffuse fear about the MPD diagnosis. In addition, MPD peer networks can also help MPD patients find a qualified therapist.

Alcohol and Substance Abuse Groups

Now that we are beginning to know more about MPD, it is becoming evident that many of these patients are alcohol and/or substance abusers or have such a personality in their system (Peabody 1985). In fact, this often serves as a cover for some of their bizarre behavior that is witnessed by others. This behavior is typically attributed to the effects of drugs or alcohol.

Several clinicians have observed that MPD patients have an unusually high tolerance for medication and can often consume amounts that would render most normal individuals unconscious (Barkin et al. 1985 [see also Chapter 5 in this book]; Braun 1983; Kluft 1985). These clinicians have recommended that medication be used very cautiously and that phenothiazines are contraindicated in the primary treatment of MPD. From these observations, one can infer that many MPD patients attempt to anesthesize or self-medicate. If this issue is not addressed in treatment, it is possible to have a fully integrated patient who is still an alcoholic or a substance abuser.

Groups such as Alcoholics Anonymous or Narcotics Anonymous are useful adjuncts to the overall treatment rationale. The primary therapist should contract with the patient about which personalities will attend the group meetings. In addition, contracting with other personalities is useful in preventing the substance-abusing personalities from damaging the body.

Leisure Activity of Special Talent Groups

Multiple personality disorder has often been called a "secret disorder" because it is extremely difficult to diagnose (Braun and Sachs 1985). These patients have spent most of their lives hiding from both themselves and others. In this regard, any social connection the therapist can help the MPD patient make is helpful. Special talent groups or leisure activity groups provide an additional network for healthy interpersonal contact. Many MPD patients are extremely creative, and these special activity groups help patients express their talents.

Vocational Counselors

The use of vocational counseling can sometimes be helpful after the primary treatment has progressed to the point at which the MPD patient is capable of functioning effectively in his or her social environment. Vocational counselors can help the MPD patient market existing skills, help the patient to clarify vocational interests, and identify where the patient can receive suitable occupational training. Initially, the MPD patient is best suited for employment in a low-stress situation, but as therapy progresses he or she may be able to handle more challenging work environments. Many MPD patients are able to lead very productive lives in high-prestige jobs.

Tutorial Groups

Tutorial groups are often useful in helping MPD patients learn remedial academic skills they missed while dissociating in school. These groups are for educational purposes only, and it is not necessary for anyone else in the group to know that the patient is suffering from MPD.

24-Hour Hotlines

Many MPD patients report difficulty sleeping. This is typically because many childhood abuses occurred late at night when the child was thought to be sleeping. In addition, many abuses are restimulated through dreams. These nightmares often leave the patient in a state of terror which makes sleeping impossible. Twenty-four-hour hotlines are useful in this regard because an empathic listener is guaranteed. The primary therapist may give the MPD patient the phone number of a 24-hour hotline for this purpose.

SUMMARY

In summary, th 3-P model of MPD can be useful in identifying how the positive effects of social support systems can be adjunctively incorporated into the overall treatment plan for MPD. These systems help mitigate these factors that perpetuate MPD, establish healthy social interactions, and reduce the likelihood of therapist burnout. Such interventions can include marital and family therapy as well as the services of various social agencies. For example, various agencies deal with parenting issues, incest and child abuse, assertiveness training, alchohol and substance abuse problems, vocational issues, and educational remediation. Other support networks include the clergy, peer networks, and 24-hour hotlines. It is hoped that therapists working with MPD patients will learn to identify and make better use of all of these social support systems in their communities.

REFERENCES

Abused and Neglected Child Reporting Act. PA 81-1077, effective July 1 1980. Illinois Department of Children and Family Services

American Psychiatric Association: Diagnostic and Statistical Manual of Mental Disorders (Third Edition). Washington, DC, American Psychiatric Association, 1980

Bandura A: Social Learning Theory. Englewood Cliffs, NJ, Prentice Hall, 1977

Barkin RL, Braun BG, Kluft RP: The dilemma of drug therapy for multiple personality disorders, in Dissociative Disorders 1985; Proceedings of the Second International Conference on Multiple Personality/Dissociative States. Edited by Braun BG. Chicago, Rush University, 1985

Braun BG: Psychophysiologic phenomena in multiple personality and hypnosis. Am J Clin Hypn 26:124–137, 1983

Braun BG: The transgenerational incidence of dissociation and multiple personality disorder: a preliminary report, in Childhood Antecedents of Multiple Personality. Edited by Kluft RP. Washington, DC, American Psychiatric Press, 127–150, 1985

Braun BG, Sachs RG: The development of multiple personality disorder: predisposing, precipitating, and perpetuating factors, in Childhood Antecedents of Multiple Personality. Edited by Kluft RP. Washington, DC, American Psychiatric Press, 37–64, 1985

Brown G, Birley J, Wing J: Influence of family life in the course of schizophrenic disorders: a replication. Br J Psychiatry 121:241–258, 1972

Cutrona C: Social support and stress in the transition to parenthood. Journal of Abnormal Psychology 93:378–390, 1984

Fagan J, McMahon P: Incipient multiple personality in children: four cases. J Nerv Ment Dis 172:26–36, 1984

Finney JW, Moos RH: Characteristics and prognoses of alcoholics who become moderate drinkers and abstainers after treatment. Journal of Studies of Alcoholism, 42, 94–105, 1981

Kempe R, Kempe C: Child Abuse. Cambridge, MA, Harvard University Press, 1978

Kluft RP: Treatment of multiple personality disorder, in Symposium on Multiple Personality. Edited by Braun BG. Psychiatr Clin North Am 7:9–30, 1984a

Kluft RP: Multiple personality in childhood, in Symposium on Multiple Personality. Edited by Braun BG. Psychiatr Clin North Am 7:21–34, 1984b

Kluft RP: The treatment of multiple personality disorder: current concepts. Directions in Psychiatry (Volume 5). Edited by Flach FF. New York, Heatherleigh, 1985

Kluft RP, Braun BG, Sachs RG: Multiple personality, intrafamial abuse, and family psychiatry. Int J Fam Psychiatry 5:283–301, 1985

Kramer C: The Theoretical Position: Diagnostic and Therapeutic Implications in the Beginning Phase of Family Treatment. Chicago, Kramer Foundation, 1968

Peabody LK: Alcoholism/chemical dependency: implications in the treatment of multiple personality disorder, in Dissociative Disorders 1985; Proceedings of the Second International Conference on Multiple Personality/Dissociative States. Edited by Braun BG. Chicago, Rush University, 1985

Putnam FW, Post RM, Guroff JJ, et al: 100 cases of multiple personality disorder (New Research Abstract No. 77). Presented at the annual meeting of the American Psychiatric Association, New York, 1983

Schultz RK, Braun BG, Kluft RP: Creativity and the imaginary companion phenomenon: prevalence and phenomenology in MPD, in Dissociative Disorders 1985; Proceedings of the Second International Conference on Multiple Personality/Dissociative States. Edited by Braun BG. Chicago, Rush University, 1985

Wilbur CB: Multiple personality and child abuse. Psychiatr Clin North Am 7:3–8, 1984

9

The Treatment of Multiple Personality: State of the Art

Frank W. Putnam, M.D.

9

The Treatment of Multiple Personality: State of the Art

Multiple personality disorder (MPD), as a distinct clinical entity, can be traced back to the 17th century (Bliss 1980). The history of the disorder shows a cyclic waxing and waning in the numbers of clinical case reports (Ellenberger 1970; Sutcliffe and Jones 1962). The reasons for these fluctuations in the apparent numbers of recognized cases are complex and have been ascribed to several factors: 1) the decline in the use of hypnosis in psychiatry (Braun 1984), 2) reaction to charges that the clinicians who diagnosed MPD were duped by their patients or even were charlatans colluding with their patients in deceiving others (Ellenberger 1970; Rosenbaum 1980), and 3) the increasing popularity of the diagnosis of schizophrenia over the last 60 years (Rosenbaum 1980). Currently we are again experiencing a dramatic increase in the numbers of patients receiving the diagnosis of MPD (Boor 1982; Braun 1984b; Greaves 1980; Kluft 1984c).

A full understanding of the state of the art in diagnosis and

The author would like to gratefully acknowledge the contributions and comments of Richard J. Loewenstein, M.D., Richard J. Wyatt, M.D., and Juliet J. Guroff.

treatment of MPD requires that one view our present state of knowledge from a historical perspective. Bliss (1980), in his article on 14 cases of MPD, credited Paracelsus with the first report of a case of 1646. By the 19th century, case reports became common and included some excellent descriptions of treatment, most notably Despine's work with "Estelle" in 1836 (Ellenberger 1970; Kluft 1984d). During the early part of the 19th century, Benjamin Rush and others investigated and described cases of dissociation and multiple personality (Carlson 1981, 1984). At the turn of the century, Morton Prince (Prince 1906, 1975) and William James (Ellenberger 1970; Taylor 1983) were among the notable researchers who devoted considerable attention to the phenomena of dissociation and multiple personality.

For a number of reasons well reviewed by Ellenberger (1970) and Rosenbaum (1980), the diagnosis of MPD fell into disrepute shortly after the turn of the century and the number of reports plunged (Rosenbaum 1980). In a thoughtful analysis of the historical context in which this decline occurred, Rosenbaum suggested that the replacement of "dementia praecox" with the term "schizophrenia," introduced by Bleuler in 1910, may have contributed to the misdiagnosis and consequent mistreatment of MPD patients. He noted that Bleuler encouraged this trend when he stated that "all cases so diagnosed [hysterical psychoses] by others differed in no ways from other schizophrenias" (Rosenbaum 1980, p. 1385). Multiple personality disorder patients are still trying to escape from what Rosenbaum termed the "schizophrenia net," as numerous case reports, reviews, and case series document (Bliss 1980; Boor 1982; Greaves 1980; Kluft 1984c; Putnam et al. 1986).

Although "The Three Faces of Eve" (Thigpen and Cleckley 1954) was an important case report that served to redirect attention to the syndrome after a long absence from the clinical literature, the media representations of Eve presented a stereotype of MPD patients that made recognition of actual cases more difficult for many professionals without other sources of information about MPD. The seminal case of "Sybil" (Schreiber 1973), with its clear description of phenomenology and treatment, facilitated recognition of MPD patients and began the current dramatic increase in the numbers of diagnosed cases. It is a statement about the tenor of the times that the eloquent description of Cornelia Wilbur's successful treatment of Sybil that was presented in a professional symposium was deliberately excluded from publication in the proceedings of that symposium and had to be reported in the lay press by Schreiber (1973).

In the face of professional indifference or outright hostility to the diagnosis of MPD and the near impossibility of getting articles on MPD published in professional journals, clinicians interested in these patients were forced to create other forums for the presentation and exchange of ideas on diagnosis and treatment. Kluft (1985d) described the development of an "oral literature" on MPD, which occurred in conjunction with the organization of courses, workshops, and newsletters by the modern pioneers in the treatment of this disorder. As is the case with all oral literatures, the authorship of individual contributions to the body of knowledge becomes blurred with time. Braun formalized the oral tradition in 1984, by instituting the annual International Conference on Multiple Personality/Dissociative States, sponsored by Rush-Presbyterian-St. Luke's Medical Center.

The inclusion of a dissociative disorders category and the formal recognition of MPD as a discrete clinical entity in the *Diagnostic and Statistical Manual of Mental Disorders (Third Edition) (DSM–III* American Psychiatric Association 1980) has redressed the prior denial of the diagnosis. In response to this formal legitimization, clinical literature on MPD and other forms of dissociation has grown rapidly. During 1983 and 1984 four journals devoted special issues to the disorder (Braun 1983a, 1984a; Kluft 1984a; Orne 1984). Kluft's seminal edition on childhood MPD (Kluft 1985a), the present book, and other work yet to come are a testament to the efforts of the modern pioneers and experts to share their knowledge of MPD with others in the mental health and medical professions.

THE CURRENT STATE OF CLINICAL KNOWLEDGE

As with most technical endeavors, the published information on the diagnosis and treatment of MPD lags behind the practice of the art. Cursory examination of the recent literature reveals a wide range of different treatment modalities advocated as primary therapeutic interventions for MPD. In just the last decade, articles have appeared describing the use of psychoanalysis (Lampl-de-Groot 1981; Lasky 1978; Marmer 1980), hypnosis (Braun 1980, 1984d; Horevitz 1983; Howland 1975; Kluft 1982, 1983), behavior modification (Caddy 1985; Price and Hess 1979), family therapy (Beale 1978; Davis and Osherson 1977; Kluft et al. 1985; Levenson and Berry 1983), group therapy (Caul 1984; Coons and Bradley 1985), amobarbital-facilitated psychotherapy (Hall et al. 1975), and anticonvulsant medication (Mesulam 1981; Schenk and Bear 1981). A closer look at the literature reveals that most of these treatment recommendations are complementary or adjunctive rather than mutually exclusive interventions. Clinical descriptions and recommendations indicate that most MPD patients share a constellation of symptoms. The variety of therapeutic interventions advocated by modern therapists reflects the diversity of theoretical orientations and professional training being applied to treatment of MPD.

Prior to the work of Ralph Allison (Allison and Schwarz 1980), the literature on the treatment of MPD consisted primarily of single case reports and a few reviews based on these reports. Coons (1984) observed that the latter often included cases that would not meet current *DSM-III* criteria. Treatment recommendations were often made on the basis of a clinician's experience with a single case, frequently the clinician's first MPD patient, who often was not seen for more than a few sessions. In the absence of better data, these early impressionistic recommendations served to orient neophytes to some of the more salient clinical findings and treatment issues. Unfortunate generalizations, however, were sometimes offered on the basis of this very limited experience (Kluft 1985a). As Kluft observed, MPD patients are a very diverse group and it is not surprising that contradictory assertions would accumulate in the literature as a result of this narrow perspective. The problem of inappropriate generalizations from limited data continues to plague the study of MPD.

Recently, a considerable body of clinical knowledge has formed based on experience with relatively large numbers of MPD patients. Pioneering work by Eugene Bliss, Bennett Braun, David Caul, Philip Coons, George Greaves, Richard Kluft, Roberta Sachs, David Spiegel, and Cornelia Wilbur, to name only a few of the contributing clinicians, has provided a firm foundation upon which to base diagnostic and treatment guidelines. A point-by-point review of the current clinical knowledge of MPD is beyond the scope of this paper. Instead, I present a summary of the evidence that suggests that the clinical knowledge we have acquired on the diagnosis and treatment of MPD is a useful and valid knowledge.

Replication of Findings

Independent replication of findings, a basic principle of the scientific method, provides the first line of evidence that our clinical knowledge of MPD is reliable and valid. The history of MPD is filled with the empirical discovery and independent rediscovery of the same findings by clinicians who have been unaware of each other's work. Kluft has pointed out that Despine's treatment recommendations, made 150 years ago, have been reaffirmed as basic treatment principles in modern cases (Kluft 1985b). A comparison of videotaped therapeutic behaviors among experienced MPD therapists led Braun and others to conclude that the clinical realities of working with MPD patients elicit common responses in therapists irrespective of these therapists' theoretical orientations (Kluft 1985d). The principle of independent replication of clinical findings is best exemplified in the realm of diagnosis and symptomatology. A comparison of data obtained from reviews of the literature (Boor 1982; Greaves 1980), patient series diagnosed by a single clinician (Bliss 1980, 1984a, 1984b; Horevitz and Braun 1984; Kluft 1984e), and a survey of independent cases in treatment across North America (Putnam et al. 1986) all show a high degree of agreement for the frequency of specific psychiatric and medical symptoms and the phenomenology of the multiplicity (Bliss 1984a; Putnam et al. 1986).

A second example of the independent replication of findings is the development of predictor lists for the signs and symptoms of MPD in children and adolescents. Three separate but highly overlapping lists were developed by clinicians working with child MPD patients (Elliott 1982; Fagan and McMahon 1984; Kluft 1984). Although these lists were shared among the investigators in a prepublication phase of development, they had been derived from independent clinical work.

More evidence of replication is the verification by systematic studies of the clinical observation and theoretical predictions made by therapists working with MPD patients. A good example is the confirmation by systematic studies with appropriate control groups of the high degree of hypnotic susceptibility reported in MPD patients by their therapists. Clinicians have often commented on the high degree of hypnotizability of MPD patients (Alexander 1956; Beahrs 1982; Bliss 1980; Bowers and Brecher 1955; Braun 1980; Howland 1975; Kluft 1982; Lipton 1943; Morton and Toma 1964). Bliss demonstrated in a series of reports (1983, 1984a, 1984b) that MPD patients have a significantly higher hypnotic susceptibility than do control subjects.

A final example of the systematic replication of earlier clinical observations is the recurrent independent finding that MPD patients are significantly more likely to have a childhood history of severe trauma, usually some form of child abuse, than are other psychiatric patients. The linkage of the development of MPD to childhood trauma has been widely noted by therapists working with these patients (Bliss 1980; Boor 1982; Braun and Sachs 1985; Brende and Rinsley 1981; Coons 1984; Greaves 1980; Putnam et al. 1986; Saltman and Solomon 1982; Schreiber 1973; Wilbur 1984, 1985). Coons (1985) found that MPD patients are significantly more likely to have a childhood history of physical and sexual abuse than are a control group of age- and sex-matched psychiatric patients.

Pragmatic Validation

A second line of evidence that indicates that our current base of knowledge of diagnosis and treatment is valid and useful comes in the form of pragmatic results. It works! And it works in a population of patients for whom other standard psychiatric interventions have failed miserably. Many MPD patients have experienced prolonged courses of treatment under misdiagnoses like schizophrenia, bipolar and unipolar affective disorders, personality disorders (particularly borderline), anxiety disorders, and temporal lobe epilepsy (Bliss 1980; Kluft 1984c; Putnam et al. 1986). The NIMH survey found that MPD patients averaged almost seven years in the mental health system for symptoms referable to MPD before the correct diagnosis was made. Most of these patients received three or four other psychiatric and/or neurologic diagnoses during this period (Putnam et al. 1986). In fact, refractoriness to standard psychiatric interventions for a given diagnosis has been cited as a signal that should increase a clinician's index of suspicion for the possibility of MPD (Putnam et al. 1984).

Our current knowledge about the treatment of MPD is derived exclusively from the work of clinicians, often in nonacademic settings, who have been sticking it out in the trenches with these complex and difficult patients. Their acceptance or rejection of specific techniques is based on the success or failure of these interventions. Their conviction of the correctness of their methods comes from seeing these patients dramatically improve and in many cases actually get 'well' when all other treatments have failed. This form of proof, although very difficult to document systematically for any single clinician, is nonetheless very convincing to the therapist who observes it in his or her patient.

Citing the oral literature, Kluft (1985d) stated that there is "increasing agreement that the prognosis for most patients with MPD is quite optimistic if intense and prolonged treatment from experienced clinicians can be made available" (p. 3). The best evidence for a good outcome with current treatment recommendations comes from Kluft's own meticulous work. In a series of reports (1984e; see also Chapter 2 in this monograph), he describes the outcome of a large cohort of MPD patients diagnosed by rigorous criteria and aggressively followed up on over several years. The evidence indicates that sustained unification of personality can be achieved and maintained in MPD patients, even in the face of significant life stress.

Similarity of Models of Multiple Personality Disorder

A line of evidence indicating that we are converging on a better understanding of MPD comes from the development of similar or complementary theories and models of the disorder. In this book, Braun, Kluft, and Spiegel all discuss their models of MPD (see Chapters 1, 4, and 3, respectively). Braun views MPD from the perspective of predisposing, precipitating, and perpetuating factors necessary for the development and maintenance of MPD. Kluft has developed a four-factor theory of MPD, and Spiegel has conceptualized MPD as a form of posttraumatic stress disorder. A detailed comparison of these models by the reader will show that all of these models attempt to account for a similar set of observations and facts.

The current state of our knowledge of MPD rests in large part on the strong consensus on diagnosis and treatment reached in the oral literature among clinicians with widely ranging theoretical orientations and professional training. This information is rapidly making its way into print and will increasingly become available to the larger professional community. From a historical perspective, the generation of an oral literature was a necessary and understandable response to the prior professional indifference or hostility that excluded the modern pioneers from access to the usual professional forums. The currently emerging clinical literature provides strong evidence in the form of independent replication that there is a core set of symptoms and behaviors shared by most MPD patients. There is also a consensus that childhood trauma, particularly child abuse, is a general historical feature of these patients and most probably is a significant etiological factor in the development of MPD. The published treatment studies to date agree with the oral literature and indicate that when properly diagnosed and treated, MPD patients have a generally good prognosis.

THE NEXT STEP: MORE SYSTEMATIC STUDY OF TREATMENT OF MULTIPLE PERSONALITY DISORDER

Therapists and investigators of MPD find themselves in a situation that has occurred many times before in the history of medicine. Sir Bradford Hill (1962), in his classic text on medical research, eloquently summed up the nature of this predicament.

> Personal observations of a handful of patients, acutely made and accurately recorded by the masters of clinical medicine have been, and will continue to be, fundamental to the progress of medicine. Of that, however statistically minded this age may be or may become, there can be no doubt whatever. What can happen, what does exist, quite regardless of the frequency of occurrence and irrespective of causation of association, may be observed on a sample of one.
>
> The field of medical observation . . . is often narrow in the sense that no one doctor will treat many cases in a short space of time; it is wide in the sense that a great many doctors may

each treat a few cases. Thus, with a somewhat ready assumption of cause and effect and, equally, a neglect of the laws of chance, the literature becomes filled with conflicting cries and claims, assertions and counterassertions. It is thus, for want of an adequately controlled test, that various forms of treatment have in the past become unjustifiably, even sometimes harmfully established in everyday medical practice. (p. 3)

The next step necessary to advance the current state of knowledge of MPD is the initiation of more systematic studies of the disorder using standardized and accepted methodology. This has long been recognized by the pioneers of MPD. Kluft, whose carefully documented treatment series (1984e) provides much of the current published evidence for the efficacy of psychotherapy augmented by hypnotherapy in MPD, has been in the forefront of advocating more objective research on different treatment approaches to MPD. The current existence of open studies of treatment of MPD is, however, a tradition practiced by every specialty area of medicine. Levine observed (1981a) that virtually all early trials of a new therapy are performed in an uncontrolled manner. In fact, in the past many important medical therapies, for example the use of penicillin for bacterial infections, were accepted solely on the basis of open clinical trials. Present professional standards, however, require more proof than in the past.

Reasons for Standardization of Investigations of Treatment of Multiple Personality Disorder

Standardized and controlled investigations of MPD are desirable for several reasons. First, we need to know what the treatments of choice are for MPD patients. Although we believe that the cumulative experience and relative consensus of experienced therapists have defined a set of strategies and identified many unique aspects of the treatment of MPD, many areas of uncertainty remain that will require a more systematic evaluation.

A second compelling reason to pursue systematic investigations of different treatment modalities is that this form of proof is necessary to convince most professionals who are not familiar with the field of the superiority of one form of intervention over another. Systematic studies are required to establish the efficacy of psychiatric therapy for other psychiatric disorders, and MPD will be held accountable to the same standard. In addition, it is important that the mental health disciplines have the information derived from such studies to serve as a standard to judge professional conduct. For professional, ethical, and legal reasons, we need to know what constitutes acceptable treatment.

A third reason for pursuing standardized studies is economics. Insurance companies and other third-party payment sources will demand evidence of the efficacy of specific treatment interventions before they will provide reimbursement for these treatments. Psychotherapy augmented by hypnosis is the treatment of choice on the basis of current knowledge of MPD (Kluft 1985d). In most cases, medications are useful only as limited adjunctive interventions to control secondary symptoms or concurrent disorders (see Chapter 5; also Kluft 1984b, 1985d). Inpatient treatment has utility, but it is limited; most therapists strive for an outpatient setting (Putnam et al. 1986). Yet many third-party payment agencies are more willing to fund medication and hospital-based treatment than outpatient psychotherapy. Systematic studies will be necessary to establish the cost effectiveness of inpatient and/or outpatient psychotherapy-oriented treatment of MPD.

A fourth reason to undertake standardized investigations of the treatment of MPD concerns the need of the field to establish credibility within the professional community. The history of MPD is filled with examples in which hard-won clinical knowledge has been discounted or ignored because the phenomenology associated with the patients' alternate personalities strains credulity. Systematic studies of these patients conducted at a number of sites would significantly enhance the credibility of the disorder in certain circles.

The final and most far-reaching and important reason for standardization of MPD treatment investigations is that a better understanding of MPD may possibly provide an important window into areas of psychosomatic medicine, the development of personality, mechanisms of learning and memory, and the nature of consciousness (Putnam, 1984a). It is a widely shared observation among experienced MPD therapists that MPD patients often exhibit profound psychophysiological shifts when they switch personalities and may manifest personality-specific physiological responses (Braun 1983; Putnam 1984a; Putnam et al. 1986; see also Chapter 5 in this book). The scientific study of MPD can also be anticipated to provide us with many insights into the mechanisms of other pathological shifts in state of mind such as occur in manic-depressive illness, episodic dyscontrol syndromes, and the flashbacks and abreactions that can occur in traumatic neuroses.

What Is Required for a More Systematic Approach to Treatment of Multiple Personality Disorder?

In general, controlled clinical studies require that important variables be identified and controlled for in a systematic fashion. The treatment protocols under evaluation need to be carefully specified and carried out. Most current clinical trial designs require the randomized assignments of patients to different treatment groups for comparison of the efficacy of two or more modalities. In addition, single-blind and double-blind methodology is preferred to ensure objectivity in the collection of data. Frequently some form of crossover from active treatment to placebo is incorporated to control for often potent placebo effects.

Difficulties in Systematization of Multiple Personality Disorder Treatment Investigations

When one begins to contemplate the design of studies to compare the efficacy of two or more treatment modalities in MPD patients, for example, hypnotherapy versus neuroleptic medications, it quickly becomes apparent that even simple studies are difficult to do. There are a large number of potentially important variables to be controlled. These include the usual demographic factors such as age, sex, socioeconomic status; variables such as concurrent medical, neurological, or other psychiatric pathology; and the effects of concurrent or prior treatment. In addition, one needs to control for many of the variables and dynamics unique to MPD. These include such relatively unknown quantities as patient type (for example, simple versus complex polyfragmented cases (see Chapter 1), presence or absence of specific types of alternate personalities such as "internal self-helpers" (Allison and Schwarz 1980), and age at the time of therapeutic intervention. This last variable has been identified as important by therapists working with child and adolescent MPD patients (Kluft 1985c). The large number of variables that may prove to be important in such studies requires researchers to think in terms of multivariate statistical designs, which in turn requires a large sample size in order to have discriminative power.

Many other difficulties exist in working with MPD patients that can be fully appreciated only by those who have had the opportunity to work with an MPD patient or two (Putnam 1984b). They produce complex transference and countertransference interactions and can wreak havoc on any research team or hospital ward that is not well informed and prepared. Anecdotal reports suggest that as a group, MPD patients have a heightened sensitivity to medication side effects and often exhibit marked placebo responses to any intervention (Kluft 1984b). They are exquisitely sensitive to milieu issues and can have strong negative reactions to seemingly innocuous stimuli that in fact are highly charged idiosyncratic conditioned cues.

One might also anticipate that experienced clinicians, who are the most qualified to participate in treatment studies, would not desire to take part in any study that offers a form of treatment that they believe to be ineffective or detrimental to their patients. A further factor compounding the difficulty of performing systematic studies with MPD patients is the lack of any financial base of support. There has never been a single federal grant awarded to support research on MPD, and investigators of MPD are going to have to break into a highly competitive funding arena during a period when support for research in all areas of mental health is declining.

The dilemma at this point is that although systematic investigations into MPD are highly desirable, they are also exceedingly difficult to accomplish. The difficulties lie in the lack of resources available to investigators, in the complex multivariate design issues, and in the pragmatic difficulties of working with these patients in a research setting.

A Potential Solution to the Difficulties of Systematization of Multiple Personality Disorder Treatment Investigations: A Multicenter Approach

One only has to consider the millions of dollars and hundreds of thousands of labor hours expended in investigating psychiatric disorders such as schizophrenia and affective illness to realize that practical strategies for the research of MPD must be simple and modest. In the foreseeable future, only a small fraction of the resources now invested in the study of schizophrenia and affective disorders will be available to researchers of MPD. Consequently, we will have to devise study designs that take maximum advantage of what is currently or readily available.

We have to restrain our natural inclination to go for a "knockout blow" in studying MPD and begin by dividing the larger questions into a series of smaller, more easily testable questions. Parallel pursuit of answers to a sequence of small, carefully chosen questions by clinicians and investigators collaborating at a number of independent sites can effect a larger perspective on MPD. This strategy permits accumulation of a much larger sample size than could be accommodated by any single site. When carefully coordinated, this strategy also enables us to include a range of control groups to control for the many potentially relevant variables.

I propose that we begin planning a series of small, cooperative, multicenter studies on the phenomenology, treatment, and outcome of MPD. When well executed, several small-scale studies, each addressing specific but overlapping questions, can provide a great deal more information than can one or two larger studies, assuming that the latter could even be attempted given the current limitation of resources. A series of coordinated small-scale studies would provide the following advantages:

1. A larger cumulative sample size than could be achieved by a single conventional study.
2. Incorporation of a number of different control groups would allow for the identification and control of many more variables than could be handled in a single conventional study.
3. Comparable data on patient and control groups could be exchanged among investigators for comparison of results.
4. Testing, replication, validation, and cross-validation of a number of measures and scales for the diagnosis and outcome of MPD would be possible.
5. Separate funding sources and local resources could be used for each study. Because the amounts would be less than that

required for one or two larger studies, they could be more
easily raised.

6. Replication of the findings of one group by other centers
   could be rapid. Networking among investigators would by-
   pass the long delay that follows collection, analysis, and publication by one group and the incorporation of that
   information into the planning and implementation of studies
   by other researchers. In addition, networking permits the
   coordination of studies so that investigators are not need-
   lessly duplicating each other's efforts.
7. The training of a core group of researchers familiar with
   MPD who could then initiate other important investigations,
   including studies into the nature of alternate personalities
   and their role in mind/body problems.

Implementation of a multicenter approach would require a
high level of cooperation among participating investigators and
would necessitate the establishment of a centralized coordination mechanism. Participants would be linked by a formal com-
puter network, which would allow for the exchange of
information and data. Such networks have well-established
precedents in industry and are being increasingly implemented
in the sciences. Clinical material, necessary for the standardization of diagnosis and rating instruments, can be exchanged
by videocassette. Already a number of units or centers are in
place or planned that specialize in the diagnosis and treatment
of MPD and related dissociative disorders. These sites could
provide the initial nodes for this network. Presently, the field
of dissociative disorders is small enough that most of the leading
clinicians and investigators are well acquainted with each other,
and many have already established working relationships. This
proposal would take advantage of these existing alliances.

The implementation of these studies must be staged so that
they build on each other in a cross-sectional and longitudinal
fashion. If one accepts Kluft's (1984e) rule that "no multiple is
considered to be successfully integrated until two years and
three months after the final integration" (p. 13), one can immediately see that treatment studies will need to stretch out
over many years to effectively measure outcome. Given that the
average treatment length for adult MPD patients is thought to
be about three to five years, such studies would then require

roughly five to seven years to complete. It is unrealistic to expect any beginning research group to embark on a study that will at best show results in five years.

Instead, each investigational site can participate in a series of short-term studies that would over time also accumulate a cohort of patients for long-term outcome comparisons. This would allow each of the participating centers to develop its local resources and to integrate the research effort into ongoing treatment programs at its own rate. On the national level, this spaced start-up sequence would provide an opportunity to develop and test the coordination of clinical measures and the exchange of information and data. As these tasks become more routine, new sites could be brought online increasingly rapidly, and more ambitious goals could be set.

An Example of a Multicenter Study

The following scenario, although obviously utopian in some respects, is one example of how such a multicenter project might work. The initial focus of the study would be the collection of data on the presenting symptoms, past history, and clinical phenomenology (for example, numbers and types of alternate personalities, concurrent psychiatric disorders such as substance abuse). Sufficient information exists about these questions to stimulate the formulation of a number of specific hypotheses and aid in the identification of potentially important variables. The project should begin with what we know the most about and proceed from there. Hypothetical Study Site A might be a clinic located in a major East Coast metropolitan area, Study Site B might be a clinic in the rural South, Study Site C might be a Midwest state institution for chronic inpatients, and Study Site D might be a West Coast penal institution.

All investigators would use a set of agreed-upon diagnostic criteria, symptom checklists, and standardized rating scales. Standardization of diagnosis and ratings could be done across study sites using the videotape methodology developed by the National Institute of Mental Health Collaborative Study on the Psychobiology of Depression which successfully used a multicenter approach. Andreasen et al. (1982) found a very high degree of intercenter reliability on diagnosis and clinical phenomenology using the videotape assessment techniques pioneered in this study. Additional measures of special interest to specific investigators, for example hypnotic susceptibility, could be used at one or more sites. The control groups used by each site would differ along some variables and could be equated on others.

All four sites would then survey their population and analyze their data on patients and controls. Each group would have its own publishable study and could draw on the data of other groups for comparison of results. On certain measures, the data of another group might be directly included in the analysis of a given group's results. In addition, the project as a whole would analyze the overall results of the pooled data.

Some subset of the patients included in the initial studies of clinical presentation and phenomenology would continue to be involved in ongoing therapy at each of the study sites, providing the patient sample for the outcome studies. The first treatment modality outcome studies would not require a randomized clinical design. It is generally accepted that institution of a randomized clinical research design is ethical only when an investigator can state an honest null hypothesis (Levine 1981b). In other words, the investigator must be able to show that there is no scientifically valid reason to predict that Treatment A is superior to Treatment B for the group of patients under study. Given the accumulated clinical knowledge with MPD patients, one could not, for example, state an honest null hypothesis for the comparison of psychotherapy and neuroleptics.

Clinicians who are doing research in cancer therapy often face a similar problem. One solution has been the use of historical control group designs. In these studies, patients are offered the treatment that is believed to be the best and their outcome is compared with that of patients who were previously treated for the same disease, whether or not the results of the latter group were obtained in the course of organized trials (Cowan 1982). This design allows an assessment of the relative efficacy of a treatment modality. Other control group options are also available. Waiting-list controls have been used in some psychotherapy studies (O'Leary and Borkovec 1978). The use of dropouts, although they represent a self-selected subpopulation, can still provide useful information on the natural course and outcome of untreated MPD. One advantage of a multicenter study approach is that a national data base of dropouts and waiting-list controls can be established upon which all project participants could draw.

The comparison of treatment modalities in this first round of studies would entail the careful characterization of the therapy offered at each study site. Methodology for doing this has been developed by psychotherapy researchers and can be readily adapted to MPD research. This approach would allow each investigative team to offer the treatment they believe to be the best for their patients. No therapist would be forced to offer less than what he or she believed to be the optimum treatment. Outcome can be measured using standardized instruments and criteria adapted from other psychiatric treatment outcome studies. In addition, the unique phenomenon of fusion/integration of the alternate personalities seen in MPD treatment can be assessed using the protocols developed by Kluft (1985e). After the results from the first series of studies are available, a second round of treatment studies may be initiated in which therapeutic modalities of apparent equal benefit are assessed in true randomized and blinded fashion.

SUMMARY

Our current knowledge of the diagnosis and treatment of MPD is based on pragmatic clinical experience. This clinical knowledge has been replicated repeatedly, and a general consensus exists among clinicians experienced with these patients on the core set of symptoms, behaviors, phenomenology, etiologic factors, and treatment strategies for this disorder. We have achieved this present state of knowledge through the efforts and dedication of a small group of clinicians who have persisted in finding, treating, and reporting MPD cases, as well as in educating other mental health professionals and advocating the recognition of MPD as a legitimate clinical entity.

We are now at the point of needing more systematic investigations into MPD to advance our knowledge and provide a firm scientific, professional, and ethical foundation for the future. Given the limited resources available in this area, the standard strategies used for the study of disorders such as schizophrenia and affective illness are impractical. Instead, a series of small-scale, relatively inexpensive, multicenter investigations offers an opportunity to begin the next level of investigation into MPD. A network model of cooperation and coordination is presented that would facilitate the accumulation of a large patient sample and would allow for the controlled investigation into the large number of potentially important and confounding variables. The technology and methodology for the exchange of data and coordination of research measures is readily available, easily mastered, and inexpensive. The hope is that the initiation of a multicenter research project would ultimately produce a cadre of investigators, experienced in MPD, who could then undertake the many other interesting and potentially very important scientific questions raised by this unique disorder.

REFERENCES

Alexander VK: A case study of a multiple personality. J Abnorm Soc Psychol 52:272–276, 1956

Allison RB, Schwarz T: Minds in Many Pieces. New York, Rawson, Wade, 1980

American Psychiatric Association: Diagnostic and Statistical Manual of Mental Disorders (Third Edition). Washington, DC, American Psychiatric Association, 1980

Andreasen NC, McDonald-Scott P, Grove WM, et al: Assessment of reliability in multicenter collaborative research with a videotape approach. Am J Psychiatry 139:876–882, 1982

Beahrs JO: Unity and Multiplicity: Multilevel Consciousness of Self in Hypnosis, Psychiatric Disorder and Mental Health. New York, Brunner/Mazel, 1982

Beale EW: The use of the extended family in the treatment of multiple personality. Am J Psychiatry 135:539–542, 1978

Bliss EL: Multiple personalities: a report of 14 cases with implications for schizophrenia and hysteria. Arch Gen Psychiatry 37:1388–1397, 1980

Bliss EL: Multiple personalities, related disorders and hypnosis. Am J Clin Hypn 26:114–123, 1983

Bliss EL: A symptom profile of patients with multiple personalities, including MMPI results. J Nerv Ment Dis 172:197–202, 1984a

Bliss EL: Spontaneous self-hynosis in multiple personality disorder, in Symposium on Multiple Personality. Edited by Braun BG. Psychiatr Clin North Am 7:135–148, 1984b

Boor, M: The multiple personality epidemic: additional cases and inferences regarding diagnosis, etiology, dynamics and treatment. J Nerv Ment Dis 170:302–304, 1982

Bowers MK, Brecher S: The emergence of multiple personalities in the course of hypnotic investigation. J Clin Exp Hypn 3:188–199, 1955

Braun BG: Hypnosis for multiple personalities, in Clinical Hypnosis in Medicine, Edited by Wain HJ. Chicago, Year Book Publishers, 1980

Braun BG (Ed.): Am J Clin Hypn 26(2), October, 1983a

Braun BG: Psychophysiologic phenomena in multiple personality and hypnosis. Am J Clin Hypn 26:124–137, 1983b

Braun BG (Ed.): Symposium on Multiple Personality. Psychiatr Clin North Am 7(1), March, 1984a

Braun BG: [Foreword.] Symposium on multiple personality. Edited by Braun BG. Psychiatr Clin North Am 7:1–2, 1984b

Braun BG: Hypnosis creates multiple personality: myth or reality? Int J Clin Exp Hypn 32:191–197, 1984c

Braun BG: Uses of hypnosis with multiple personality. Psychiatric Annals 14:34–40, 1984d

Braun BG, Sachs RG: The development of multiple personality disorder: predisposing, precipitating and perpetuating factors, in Childhood Antecedents to Multiple Personality. Edited by Kluft RP. Washington, DC, American Psychiatric Press, 1985

Brende J, Rinsley D: A case of multiple personality with psychological automatisms. J Am Acad Psychoanal 9:129–151, 1981

Caddy GR: Cognitive behavior therapy in the treatment of multiple personality. Behav Modif 9:267–292, 1985

Carlson ET: The history of multiple personality in the United States: I. The beginnings. Am J Psychiatry 138:666–668, 1981

Carlson ET: The history of multiple personality in the United States: Mary Reynolds and her subsequent reputation. Bull Hist Med 58:72–82, 1984

Caul D: Group and videotape techniques for multiple personality disorder. Psychiatric Annals 14:43–50, 1984

Coons PM: The differential diagnosis of multiple personality: a comprehensive review, in Symposium on Multiple Personality. Psychiatr Clin North Am 7:51–67, 1984

Coons PM: Children of parents with multiple personality disorder, in Childhood Antecedents in Multiple Personality. Edited by Kluft RP. Washington, DC, American Psychiatric Press, 1985

Coons PM, Bradley K: Group psychotherapy with multiple personality patients. J Nerv Ment Dis 173:515–521, 1985

Cowan DH: Research on the therapy of cancer with special comment on IRB review of multiinstitutional trials, in Human Subject Research. Edited by Greenwald RA, Ryan MK, Mulvihill JE. New York, Plenum Press, 1982

Davis DH, Osherson A: The concurrent treatment of a multiple personality woman and her son. Am J Psychother 31:504–515, 1977

Ellenberger HF: The Discovery of the Unconscious. New York, Basic Books, 1970

Elliott D: State intervention and childhood multiple personality disorder. Journal of Psychiatry and Law 10:441–456, 1982

Fagan J, McMahon PP: Incipient multiple personality in children: four cases. J Nerv Ment Dis 172:26–36, 1984

Greaves GB: Multiple personality: 165 years after Mary Reynolds. J Nerv Ment Dis 168:577–596, 1980

Hall RC, Le Cann AF, Schoolar JC: Amobarbital treatment of multiple personality. J Nerv Ment Dis 161:138–142, 1975

Hill AB: Statistical methods in clinical and preventive medicine. Edinburgh, E & S Livingstone, 1962

Horevitz RP: Hypnosis for multiple personality disorder: a framework for beginning. Am J Clin Hypn 26:131–145, 1983

Horevitz PP, Braun BG: Are multiple personalities borderline? in Symposium on Multiple Personality. Edited by Braun BG. Psychiatr Clin North Am 7:69–87, 1984

Howland JS: The use of hypnosis in the treatment of a case of multiple personality. J Nerv Ment Dis 161:138–142, 1975

Kluft RP: Varieties of hypnotic interventions in the treatment of multiple personality. Am J Clin Hypn 24:230–240, 1982

Kluft RP: Hypnotherapeutic crisis intervention in multiple personality. Am J Clin Hypn 26:73–83, 1983

Kluft RP (Ed.): Psychiatric Annals 14(1): January, 1984a

Kluft RP: Aspects of the treatment of multiple personality disorder. Psychiatric Annals 14:51–57, 1984b

Kluft RP: Introduction to multiple personality disorder. Psychiatric Annals 14:51–57, 1984c

Kluft RP: Multiple personality in childhood, in Symposium on Multiple Personality. Edited by Braun BG. Psychiatr Clin North Am 7:121–134, 1984d

Kluft RP: Treatment of multiple personality disorder: a study of 33 cases, in Symposium on Multiple Personality. Edited by Braun BG. Psychiatr Clin North Am 7:9–27, 1984e

Kluft RP (Ed.): Childhood Antecedents of Multiple Personality. Washington, DC, American Psychiatric Press, 1985a

Kluft RP: Childhood multiple personality disorder: predictors, clinical findings, and treatment results, in Childhood Antecedents of Multiple Personality. Edited by Kluft RP. Washington, DC, American Psychiatric Press, 1985b

Kluft RP: Hypnotherapy of childhood multiple personality disorder. Am J Clin Hypn 27:201–210, 1985c

Kluft RP: The treatment of multiple personality disorder: current concepts, in Directions in Psychiatry (Volume 5). Edited by Flach FF. New York, Hatherleigh, 1985d

Kluft RP: Using hypnotic inquiry protocols to monitor treatment progress and stability in multiple personality disorder. Am J Clin Hypn 28:63–75, 1985e

Kluft RP, Braun BG, Sachs RG: Multiple personality, intrafamilial abuse, and family psychiatry. International Journal of Family Psychiatry 5:283–301, 1985

Lampl-de-Groot J: Notes on multiple personality. Psychoanal Q 50:614–624, 1981

Lasky R: The psychoanalytic treatment of a case of multiple personality. Psychoanal Rev 65:355–380, 1978

Levenson J, Berry S: Family intervention in a case of multiple personality. Journal of Marital and Family Therapy 9:73–80, 1983

Levine RJ: Randomized clinical trials, in Ethics and Regulation of Clinical Research. Edited by Levine RJ. Baltimore, MD, Urban and Schwarzenberg, 1981a

Levine RJ: Ethical norms and procedures, in Ethics and Regulation of Clinical Research. Edited by Levine RJ. Baltimore, MD, Urban and Schwarzenberg, 1981b

Lipton SD: Dissociated personality: a case report. Psycholanal Q 17:33–56, 1943

Marmer SS: Psychoanalysis of multiple personality. Int J Psychoanal 61:439–459, 1980

Mesulam M: Dissociated states with abnormal temporal lobe EEG. Arch Neurol 38:176–181, 1981

Morton JH, Toma E: A case of multiple personality. Am J Clin Hypn 6:216–255, 1964

O'Leary KD, Borkovec TD: Conceptual, methodological, and ethical problems of placebo groups in psychotherapy research. Am Psychol 33:821–830, 1978

Orne MT (Ed.): Int J Clin Exp Hypn 32(2), April 1984

Price J, Hess ND: Behavior therapy as a precipitant and treatment in a case of dual personality. Aust NZ J Psychiatry, 13:63–66, 1979

Prince M: Hysteria from the point of view of dissociated personality. J Abnorm Psychol 1:170–187, 1906

Prince M: Psychotherapy and multiple personality: selected essays. Edited by Hale NG Jr. Cambridge, MA: Harvard University Press, 1975

Putnam FW: The psychophysiological investigation of multiple personality disorder: a review, in Symposium on Multiple Personality. Edited by Braun BG. Psychiatr Clin North Am 7:31–39, 1984a

Putnam FW: The study of multiple personality disorder: general strategies and practical considerations. Psychiatric Annals 14:58–62, 1984b

Putnam, FW, Loewenstein RJ, Silberman EK, et al: Multiple personality in a hospital setting. J Clin Psychiatry 45:172–175, 1984

Putnam FW, Guroff JJ, Silberman EK, et al: The clinical phenomenology of multiple personality disorder: 100 recent cases. J Clin Psychiatry 47:285–293, 1986

Rosenbaum M: The role of the term schizophrenia in the decline of diagnoses of multiple personality. Arch Gen Psychiatry, 37:1383–1385, 1980

Saltman V, Solomon RS: Incest and the multiple personality. Psychol Rep 50:1127–1141, 1982

Schenk L, Bear D: Multiple personality and related dissociative phenomena in patients with temporal lobe epilepsy. Am J Psychiatry 138:1311–1316, 1981

Schreiber FR: Sybil. Chicago, Regnery, 1973

Sutcliffe, JP, Jones J: Personal identity, multiple personality and hypnosis. Int J Clin Exp Hypn 10:269–321, 1962

Taylor E: William James on Exceptional Mental States: The 1986 Lowell Lectures. Boston, University of Mass Press, 1983

Thigpen CH, Cleckley H: A case of multiple personality. Journal of Abnormal and Social Psychology 49:135–151, 1954

Wilbur CB: Multiple personality and child abuse, in Symposium on Multiple Personality. Edited by Braun BG. Psychiatr Clin North Am 7:3–8, 1984

Wilbur CB: The effect of child abuse on the psyche, in Childhood Antecedents of Multiple Personality. Edited by Kluft RP. Washington, DC, American Psychiatric Press, 1985

Index

Abreaction
  child therapy step, 100
  fusion after, 87
  in group therapy, 147, 149,
    154, 169
  integration after, 14, 92
  interpretation of, 14, 35
  in traumatic neuroses, 187
  play therapy precipitating,
    90, 92, 99–100
  quiet room, 14
  relapse likely without, 35, 38
  verbalization toward, 89
Abuse
  alcohol, 125–127, 171
  drug, 125–127, 167, 171
  marital, 167
  monitoring, 164
  patient cooperation in
    continuance, 9, 162
  physical, 8, 55, 64–66,
    68–70, 90, 162

  psychological, 67, 69, 162
  sexual, 24, 64–66, 68–70,
    139, 151
  unpredictable, 160–161
  See also Child abuse;
    Hallucinatory drugs;
    Incest
Acting out, 11, 14, 20
Alanon, 17
Alcoholics Anonymous, 17,
  171
Alternate personality (Alter)
  double bind as cause, 69
  fusion defined as absence of,
    42
  hypnosis used to contact, 12,
    89
  multiplicity of, 68, 95
  sexual abuse as cause, 64
  traits and behavior of,
    136–138
Ambivalence, 17, 20, 67